EGGS
UNSCRAMBLED

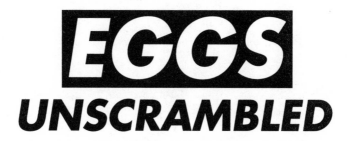

EGGS
UNSCRAMBLED

EGG FREEZING, FERTILITY, AND THE TRUTH ABOUT YOUR REPRODUCTIVE YEARS

AGNES FISCHER

Regan Arts.

NEW YORK

Regan Arts.

65 Bleecker Street
New York, NY 10012

First Regan Arts paperback edition, April 2017

Library of Congress Control Number: 2016955011

ISBN 978-1-68245-065-9

Interior design by Nancy Singer
Cover design by Richard Ljoenes

Printed in the United States of America

10 9 8 7 6 5 4 3 2 1

To my mom, Susan.
Mom, I haven't given you grandchildren yet,
but how about a book in the meantime?

a special
acknowledgment

When I started writing this book, I took our basic reproductive rights for granted. Women had relatively easy access to birth control. A woman's right to choose was solidly protected by the constitution thanks to *Roe v. Wade*. Women could control their destiny because they had agency over their own bodies. But in November 2016, America elected a president who has threatened to seriously hinder women's rights by, among other things, disavowing our reproductive freedom.

This book is about fertility and egg freezing. Many will say it's a privileged woman's issue. But I would argue it's simply a *woman's* issue, and a societal one that lives under the same umbrella as all reproductive rights. One of the many things I argue in this book is that birth control and reproductive healthcare exists on a continuum. Birth control shouldn't be defined simply as the prevention of birth, but should instead include the ability to control, or at least influence, the entirety of a woman's reproductive health and future.

So, in a politically charged environment that seems intent on taking women back 100 years, I felt compelled to acknowledge the very real threat that we all face by donating part of the proceeds of this book to Planned Parenthood—an institution whose good work largely involves preventative health care, not abortion. In fact, abortions only account for about 3 percent of the services provided to underserved women (and none of those services are funded by federal tax dollars). Thanks to organizations like Planned Parenthood, abortion rates, unwanted pregnancies, and the transmission of STDs have greatly declined (more on that later). Do we really want to see that trend reverse?

If you're a woman who believes you should be able to have babies, or *not* have babies, whenever and however she wants, join the fight to preserve our reproductive rights by supporting this book, and by supporting organizations like Planned Parenthood.

contents

foreword

by Dr. Nicole Noyes

Not many people get to say that they're in the business of helping people become parents. I'm lucky to have that privilege. I don't work miracles, but I *do* help many of the patients I see. Like all fields of medicine, in the twenty-five years I've specialized in infertility, I've witnessed a technologic explosion in the modalities that both diagnose and treat women and couples having trouble getting pregnant, so much so that today, the majority of people who seek reproductive help achieve their goals.

What has been most interesting to witness has been the drift in human reproductive trends around the globe. Specifically, in industrialized countries, the age of first birth is at an all-time high with the starting age in the US now in the latter 20s, while in Europe, Scandinavia, and parts of Asia, it has risen into the 30s. This is in spite of the fact that reproductive prime—meaning when a woman is most fertile—is age 16 to 28. Perhaps the greatest influence over this reproductive drift has been readily available, reliable birth control—most notably, the introduction of the birth control pill in the 1960s. Since that time, women (and men) have taken it upon themselves to postpone child rearing to a time they feel ready—sometimes a decade or more later than their peak fertility. This delay has led to the development of a new field of reproductive medicine known as fertility preservation.

As a female professional in a major metropolitan city who waited until 34 to conceive my first child—despite being a fertility specialist and thus having constant first-hand exposure to the trials and tribulations of trying to have a baby later in life—oocyte cryopreservation, or egg freezing, is of particular interest to me. In fact, it is the single most exciting part of my field and one that lit a fire under me in the early 2000s when I saw successes beginning to pile up at specific centers around the world. Perfecting the egg-freezing process and bringing it to the mainstream arena has been a goal for me since that time, so much so that the majority of my medical practice now includes some aspect of fertility preservation. Talking about, recommending, and seeing women through that process are regular features in my day-to-day activity. When that process comes to fruition, resulting in a child, which happens more and more as women are coming back to thaw their eggs, makes me so happy. Knowing that I can help women take charge of their fertility in this way is extraordinarily rewarding. The author of this book took charge of her own fertility in exactly that way—and I was glad to be the one to help her do so.

I first met Agnes in 2012, when she came to my office to discuss fertility. During that initial consult, Agnes disclosed that she had been married for almost two years and had been trying to get pregnant for about a year. As is my routine, prior to presenting treatment options, I probed her about her commitment to having a child; her response was that it was strong. I also asked her if she had any inkling as to why she was having trouble conceiving; always interested to hear what people *think* might be the problem and then seeing how often the perceived issue(s) turn out to be true. My take upon hearing her answers was that she knew what her issues were, being nearly 34 years old and strapped with a high-pressure, high-stress, high-travel job.

Before coming to me, Agnes had undergone some preliminary infertility testing with one of my colleagues and gynecologist-friends, Dr. Samantha Dunham, the results of which had all come back normal. I was very frank with her, informing her I would be running some additional tests but no matter what was found, the process and responsibility of fertility treatment would fall mostly on her. She would be the one would who would get poked and prodded as we tried to get her pregnant. She understood.

We then began the process of fertility treatments involving medications plus intrauterine insemination. It was then suggested to Agnes that she move on to in-vitro fertilization. She told me at that juncture that she needed to take a break from fertility treatments. What she didn't tell me until about a year later was that she also wanted to take a break from her marriage.

Agnes came back to see me in 2014, this time to talk about fertility preservation, specifically freezing her eggs. I told her I thought it was a smart move—a proactive one that she wouldn't regret. Agnes knew that at her age, fertility potential was and would continue to decline. Layered onto that was the prospect of re-entering the dating market, not easy for a mid-thirties woman. She confided that she didn't foresee suddenly and swiftly stumbling upon Mr. Right, so she wanted to put her fertility *on ice* until she figured some things out. After talking further, I came to realize the road to parenting for her didn't necessarily mean finding another husband—in fact, she talked frankly about having a child on her own and contemplated even fertilizing some of the eggs to be extracted for freezing.

Throughout Agnes' fertility journey, no matter how challenged she felt, I was impressed by her willingness to ask questions, to persevere, and to be proactive with her own situation. She even blogged about the experience—a website where she spoke openly about her egg-freezing experience with both candor and courage. After reading her book, I can say the same about the piece of literature you are currently holding in your hands.

While every patient's situation is different, a constant in my current work is the need for women to take charge of their situation so that they make thoughtful, considerate decisions regarding their own fertility journey. Agnes would—and will, in the pages that follow—show you that she did exactly that.

I say this as a doctor and as a fellow responsible, hard-working woman: It's my greatest hope that every desirous female out there will do the same.

EGGS
UNSCRAMBLED

introduction

IT IS TIME TO GET OUR HEADS OUT OF THE SAND AND INTO OUR OVARIES!

I am a thirty-something-year-old single woman who is, frankly, a little freaked out about if, when, and how I will ever have babies.

There. I said it.

Now, to be clear, I am not freaked out because I am desperate to have babies. I am freaked out because I always assumed that by my ripe old late thirties, I would have life a bit more figured out than I currently do. I took for granted that I would either have children by now, or, if not, that my *not* having children yet would be the result of some deliberate and well-thought-out choice I had made. Neither is true. So yes, I am a bit anxious about my current life situation.

This is the thing no single woman older than thirty is supposed to say. Why? Because signaling to the world that she is anxious about how her happy ending unfolds tells the world that she is a desperate creature, willing to do anything to entrap a man and strong-arm him into getting her pregnant. Saying this forbidden thing I have just said, our culture tells us, will send a man running for the hills.

I am single, yes. And yes, I wonder about what life would be like with children (and perhaps even a husband). But what I am *not* is desperate. I am—for the first time in my adult, single life—embracing my independence. My complete freedom. My lack of obligation to anyone or anything. And I would venture to guess that

1

most of my contemporaries would say the same at this point in their lives. After all, more of us are staying single longer these days, and for the simplest of reasons: because we can! As I write this book, for the first time in the history of this nation, more American adult women are single than married—and that is by choice.

It was certainly my choice, once my own marriage proved not to be the happy ending I had hoped for. I was married briefly in my early thirties, and much of that marriage was spent trying to get pregnant. In fact, it was this baby-making attempt and ultimate failure that led me to write this book, and to start speaking up (okay, maybe shouting) about fertility awareness, about understanding what happens to our bodies, what our options are to potentially preserve our fertility, and when these options come into play.

I really wanted a baby—and while I could have done what many people do, which is continue to try to get pregnant even after the marriage begins to fall apart, I was not sure I could put myself through that. Which meant I had a choice to make. I was staring at a big, fat fork in the road. On the one hand, I could continue straight down the path I had been traveling—one that headed toward offspring—because I am pretty certain my expensive, highly regarded fertility doctor would have eventually knocked me up with my then-husband's genetic material. Or I could be honest with myself and admit that he and I were heading toward divorce, and acknowledge that going down the matrimonial tubes with a little human in tow would not be fair or kind to anyone involved. All those lawyers and fights about money and deciding which of us would get the kid(s) on which holidays—it just did not sound like a fun future for any of us. And if I am really honest, I decided I would rather be single again in my thirties, without potential baby weight and baby worries, and with my body parts still firmly in place!

So I abandoned (or perhaps just put on a long pause) the baby quest and went off to find the kind of happiness that exists independently of romantic and maternal relationships. I thought it better to leave the marriage without too many battle scars—with ease, with grace, and with very little to lose. I wanted a life that did not force me to compromise at every turn. A life in which I might have a baby either with someone I could genuinely see a future with or by myself. Because while I think I do very much want to be a mom one day, I *know* I want to be happy even more.

Why am I telling you this? To assure you that you are not reading the rantings of a lunatic but rather the honest point of view of a woman who has thought about this topic an awful lot and has gone from one end of the spectrum to the other. I have experienced everything from not wanting kids to being happily married and actively trying for kids to finding myself single again, scratching my head about how I would ever have a baby, to being convinced that I should just be a single mom, to wondering if motherhood is even the right choice for me.

The point is I get it. I know life can, and does, get in the way of baby making—that a bad relationship can derail that goal, that fertility issues can throw off your plans, and that your dedication to your career can confuse the issue even further. The takeaway is this: if you think there is even the slightest chance you might one day want to be a mother, whether alone or with a man or a woman or a friend or a stranger, take a minute to think about your fertility way, way earlier than I did.

I consider myself a reasonably intelligent woman. I will not lie, I prefer E! to CNN and the "Fashion & Style" section to the rest of the *New York Times*, but in general I have it together, and when I set out to do something, it gets done. In college, I decided I wanted to work in advertising in New York City, so I moved my Southern California beach bum to the big apple right after I got my diploma while most of my friends were still recovering from graduation party alcohol poisoning. I got myself a great job and worked my way up through the male-dominated ranks of advertising. When one challenging position became boring, I moved on to the next challenging position. I ran marathons. I traveled—I went to the Middle East for fun. My successes have been punctuated by failures, sure. I am only human. But in the end, I do succeed. My highs have been punctuated by lows, but in the end, I am happy. You get the point: like most modern women who were raised thinking they could do anything the boys could do, I did, and do.

So imagine my surprise when the thing I had always taken for granted—that I would have babies one day, and that doing so would be easy—did not in fact turn out to be the case. For all my planning to accomplish things, big and small, important and meaningless, the one thing I had failed to plan for, and therefore, have failed to accomplish, is becoming a mom.

The irony, of course, is that I spent the first half of my adult life thinking *I hope I'm not pregnant.* I then moved on to the *Why am I not getting pregnant?* phase, and am now living in the land of *I hope I can still get pregnant.* (And on some days, *Do I even want to get pregnant?* I will not lie: I am still not entirely sure.)

How did this happen? And why do we live in a world of wishes and hopes rather than planning and action when it comes to getting pregnant, while we plan everything else? How did it escape me that, after a certain age, getting pregnant can be difficult? I will tell you exactly how.

First, our culture sends us faulty signals. Media-crazed and hyper-connected, we see celebrities have babies at forty-five and believe we too have plenty of time. We receive, almost by osmosis, the message that our twenties and thirties are for working hard and playing harder, and that babies come later, on that fine future day when we have finally accomplished everything we planned to. Early in my professional life, I would see women in their twenties get married or pregnant (or both). I remember thinking, *They are going to miss out on so much. They must not be very ambitious.* I had bought into the notion that one is meant to "make it" before her real life can begin. I also assumed that, like Halle Berry or Janet Jackson, I could have a baby in my forties if I chose to wait that long. I know I am not alone in having made that assumption. And I know this because, in preparation for this book, I surveyed hundreds of fierce, independent women from all over the country, and found that their knowledge was often lacking too—and that their thinking was often magical in nature.

Unfortunately, what we want and what Mother Nature allows do not always align. Our twenties are still the best time, biologically speaking, to get and stay pregnant. That is just a scientific fact. The reality is, we cannot all be Halle Berry. Those women I knew who were starting families in their early twenties were on to something, whether they knew it or not. While I do not at all regret not having babies early, and I certainly would never tell anyone they should have babies before they are ready just to outrun nature, I do believe we should all make these decisions consciously—with our eyes wide open, and armed with the most accurate information. In other words: ladies, it is time to wake up and start thinking proactively. For some reason, we seem to stay silent about fertility issues until we encounter a problem, and even then, many of us struggle through those disappointments in silence. To me, that is like talking about birth control *after* an unwanted pregnancy has occurred, or talking about protection *after* you have gotten an STD. I find it truly staggering how little most women know about their reproductive systems—and lest you think I am judging, I include myself among you. As a younger woman, aside from knowing that I got my period once a month, I could not be bothered to understand how my ovaries worked. Not entirely out of laziness, either: Because these subjects are strangely taboo among women, I did not *know* there were important things I did not know. I did not know that the health, quantity, and quality of my eggs—which is to say, my fertility—would sharply decline at a certain age. That is, I did not know that until I had already discovered I could not get pregnant without medical intervention. I needed to know that a lot sooner, as do all women.

• • •

I was thirty-three when my then-husband and I first started "trying." In the beginning, trying is actually pretty fun. (You know, because you are having a lot of sex.) But once trying becomes a monthly ritual of unsexy sex at specific (and often inconvenient) times, you will probably come to find the whole process rather trying, indeed. You and your mate may fight when he is not interested in, or is too tired for, sex at the moment you happen to be ovulating. During such fights, the conversation may devolve into him telling you he is not "a performing seal." (Nothing sexier than picturing your supposed soul mate as a large marine mammal balancing a ball on his nose.) By the time an unsuccessful year has gone by (or, if you are thirty-five or older, six months), for many people "trying" will morph into a different thing entirely: an expensive pursuit undertaken with the best doctors money can buy. Of course, that is assuming you are lucky enough to be able to pay for them.

My own fancy doctor told me that if I really wanted to get the baby-making show on the road, it was time to pump my body full of hormones and start "treatment." This is an umbrella term; "treatment" can mean a few different things. For some (including me), it means beginning a course of medication—typically Clomid, which I like to call the Crazy Pill. Clomid is a hormone that tricks your brain into thinking your body's estrogen levels are very low in order to induce the stimulation of other baby-producing hormones. The drug is taken for a few days at the beginning of the menstrual cycle, often with monitoring, so that one can bundle it with carefully timed sex. One of its fun side effects can be severe mood swings. For me, these were wild and extreme (recalling them is one of the rare occasions when I feel sympathy for my ex).

If Clomid does not work, you graduate to what I call Fertility Treatment Lite, or intrauterine insemination (IUI), of which I did one round. I have had friends refer to this as "the turkey baster method," but let me assure you, that description is misleading. A turkey baster is at least long and cylindrical and therefore penis-like, while IUI instead involves a skinny catheter full of "washed" semen that is guided, uncomfortably, past your cervix so it can enter your uterus. It is a slightly invasive procedure, and an unpleasant one. Not to mention that by the time you have reached Fertility Treatment Lite, your husband holding your hand during this process is likely the closest thing to spontaneous, not carefully timed, intimacy you have experienced in ages.

When you have gone through IUI two to three times and it has not worked, you progress on to in vitro fertilization, or IVF. I never got that far; not long after Fertility Treatment Lite failed, our marriage did too.

That was several years ago now. My lust for babies has quieted somewhat—sometimes it's entirely mute. My desperation for motherhood has been dulled, I will admit, by Xanax, copious amounts of wine, throwing myself into work, friends and travel, but also by—and this, of course, is the point of this book—a very expensive but potentially invaluable means of preserving my fertility. In short, I bought myself some time to figure out what the hell I really wanted, and how I would go about getting it.

About a year after the break-up, I shelled out nearly $20,000 and froze my eggs. Or if you want to get technical, I underwent "a cycle of oocyte cryopreservation." "Oocyte" is the medical term for an egg; "cryopreservation" means freezing cells in subzero temperatures. I am now the proud mama of twenty-eight marvelous, beautiful little potential babies, each carefully stored in the coldest of conditions. Though they have yet to be fertilized, I affectionately refer to them as "my little hatchlings."

For me, freezing my eggs felt like the right thing to do. It was the best way to quiet the voices in my head that enjoyed torturing me for not continuing on with my marriage and the fertility treatments I was undergoing with my then-husband.

I had been aware of egg freezing for some time before I did it myself, and for many years I never thought it was something I would do—mostly because I never thought I would need to. But when my marriage ended, I came to see things differently. By the time I finally pulled the trigger on the procedure, I was thirty-six. I had lived through marriage, a failed attempt at "trying," and a not-so-fun separation and the beginnings of a divorce. The point is, so much had brought me to that point, and as difficult as it was, I am glad it got me there. I would not change any of my decisions or actions. But it should not be so hard, so agonizing, to reach this decision. There should not be so many barriers for women—financial, emotional, or otherwise.

It seemed like the wisest—maybe even the *only*—choice for me. Yet I resisted it for a while. Having babies was obviously tremendously important to me, and given that I was single and thirty-five, egg freezing made a lot of sense. But I could not bring myself to freeze until I was thirty-six, a full year after I began seriously considering and investigating the procedure.

Maybe you are among the lucky people who have never been legally separated or divorced. If so, you have my envy and my admiration. Because I will be the first to tell you that neither are much fun. My separation left me insanely stressed and anxious. Not only was I just not in a good place emotionally—which makes taking on any big decision a confusing, draining, and potentially unwise prospect—I knew from experience (and many, many scientific studies) that being stressed out may not be good for one's fertility. So I knew I needed to mentally prepare myself and begin to heal emotionally before I would feel good about shelling out a ton of money to freeze my eggs.

Which leads me to the second reason I waited. Egg freezing, as I mentioned, is pretty expensive, and, annoyingly, most health insurance is absolutely useless for that procedure. So given the hefty price tag, I knew I could only afford one cycle. Which means I had to make that cycle count.

Because I wanted to wait to freeze my eggs until I was in peak health, both physically and emotionally, I spent the back half of 2014 working to get my life back together. I ate well, I exercised, I dealt with my emotions, and, ultimately, I managed to calm myself down. I cut back on alcohol—in fact, I stopped drinking entirely for the full month running up to my egg-freezing procedure, and of course I continued to abstain throughout the process, which began in January 2015.

While I felt pretty good about my decision to go forward, I knew that, being thirty-six, I was not at the primo age for egg freezing; in fact, in my opinion, I was well past it (there is a lot of debate on the right time to freeze one's eggs, which I'll discuss later). There was a part of me that felt like I was putting my energies in the wrong place, however wise I knew this decision to be. What I mean is that I kept thinking, *I should be having babies, not laying eggs.* But then again, only one of those was a viable option for me at that moment. So lay eggs I did. And it was a strange but incredible journey. Babies are miracles—we all know that. So is this procedure, even with all its complexities and variables and potential headaches. (And I encountered a few of each, believe me.)

As I underwent the procedure, I began to feel passionately that more women should know about egg freezing, and should be able to talk about it (and the issue of fertility in general) openly, without shame—and I did not see much evidence of such talk online or in books. So I started a blog, which I called Frozen Please. There, I catalogued every step of the process. I wanted to be entirely transparent: I included videos of the self-administered injections. I wrote about the medical journey, inside and out, down to every last doctor visit. I was honest about how I felt every step of the way, even when what I felt was overwhelmed or sad or exhausted by the process itself or by my various complications. I did not want other women to have to ask the same question I did at nearly every step of the "trying" process: "Why didn't anybody tell me these things?"

For example: Why did no one ever tell me that getting pregnant is not half as easy as we think it is? The statistics are staggering: 25 percent of thirty-year-old women who are trying to get pregnant naturally will not have a successful pregnancy after one year; 34 percent of thirty-five-year-old women who are trying to get pregnant naturally will not have a successful pregnancy after one year; and

56 percent of forty-year-old women who are trying to get pregnant naturally will not have a successful pregnancy after one year. And why did no one tell me that our fertility sharply declines—anywhere between a 5 and 15 percent drop per year—in our latter thirties? Or that we can only get pregnant during one extraordinarily short window each month? (I found that last one out when my gynecologist told me to buy an ovulation kit. I had never known I might need one.) If you have never had to try to get pregnant, I would be willing to bet that you, dear reader, are as surprised to hear some of these facts as I was.

One day shortly after my ex-husband and I separated, as I was in the shower in my shiny new bachelorette pad—in all likelihood washing away the hangover of the night before—a thought came to me: *Birth Control 2.0!* I was so excited about the concept, I wrote it down while still dripping wet. Birth Control 2.0 is the notion that we should put the same care and attention into managing our reproductive health and future as we put into preventing pregnancy. Birth Control 2.0 includes birth control as we commonly know it— the pill, the shot, IUDs, and so on, all centered around preventing pregnancy—but it also encompasses informed decisions about preserving fertility and navigating when, how (naturally or through assisted reproduction), where (at home or in a clinic), and with whom (a significant other or a sperm donor) we get pregnant. It is the information I wish I had had at my disposal back then, and I know many of my friends, acquaintances, and women I interviewed for this book felt the same way as they embarked upon their own fertility journeys.

Throughout the book, you will hear from several of these women—think of them as the Greek chorus chiming in now and again, putting a human face on the issue of fertility, and also infertility. These women were all kind enough to share deeply personal information with me—and now you—to help illustrate just how important it is to be aware of your reproductive potential as soon as you can be. Allow me to introduce them:

ALISON, thirty-four, is a marketing manager in San Francisco. We met after I started the blog, to which she then contributed to. She also froze her eggs. She is single, successful, whip-smart, incredibly sensitive and caring, and intensely focused on creating the life she wants. And she wants very badly to be a mom.

VICTORIA, forty-two, lives here in New York. She is a fellow advertising executive. Victoria is a single mom, and she really knows her stuff. She is fearless (deciding to embark on single motherhood is no small thing) and fierce (she does not take crap from anyone). Victoria froze her eggs in her mid-thirties but has not made use of them. And she may never need to. A couple years ago, she did a round of IUI—using her own fresh eggs—to have her lovely baby boy.

LAUREN, thirty-eight, also lives in New York, and is a freelance senior strategist. She froze her eggs three years ago, and now that she is in a long-term, committed relationship, she hopes she will not even need to use them. More and more, she is sure she wants to be a mother—for years she was only *pretty* sure—and that she wants to have her child before age forty-one.

ANA, thirty-six, is a highly accomplished lawyer. She was at a prestigious law firm in New York then Paris for several years, and now works as in-house general counsel for a highly regarded consulting firm here in New York. She is someone I have been close to nearly all my life: we are cousins. Bright, driven, and passionate, Ana has considered freezing her eggs but is still on the fence about moving forward with the procedure; she feels pretty sure that she will not wind up doing it. Though she has never tried to get pregnant, she has had her own share of challenges with her reproductive system: as a teenager, she suffered from endometriosis, a problem with the lining of the uterus, and still grapples with premenstrual dysphoric disorder (PMDD), which basically means her periods are monstrously painful and disruptive to both her physical and mental health. Though she is not all that worried about it—neither is her gynecologist—knowing she has had trouble with her reproductive organs, it has crossed her mind that getting pregnant could be more difficult than she anticipates.

KATE, forty-four, is another overachieving rock star with a tremendous intellect; she is a partner at a creative consulting firm. She got married at the very typical-for-New-York-City age of thirty-eight. She is thoughtful, self-aware, opinionated, and kind. And because life is often terribly unfair, Kate went through one of the most terrible infertility experiences imaginable. It took her years—*years*—to navigate the process of trying to conceive a child. She and her husband went through round after round of IVF. She considered pursuing adoption. Ultimately, she and her husband made use of donor eggs, which were fertilized with her husband's sperm and implanted in Kate's uterus. Today, Kate finally has her babies—twins, a boy and a girl (and they are the cutest darned little people!).

AMELIA, thirty-five, lives in San Francisco; she works in events and sponsorships there. She is single, and she froze her eggs in early 2016. Though the process was successful and relatively painless, it was still a difficult experience for her in some ways. It made Amelia angry that she had to make this choice, that getting pregnant the old-fashioned way had not happened for her. Which just goes to show how varied people's reactions to this process can be.

LAURA, thirty-three, is smart, single, gorgeous, and highly successful. She lives in New York and is a well-respected group strategy director at an advertising agency. She is a lesbian who would like to have babies one day, though not just yet. Her experience is far removed from mine, because the parameters of her potential pregnancy will be very different, but we both share the same desire to be mothers, and the same ambivalence about when and how.

HEATHER, forty—another fellow advertising executive—has spent her life working hard, and now finds herself in a high-powered, well-paying position. She did not just put off kids because she was working; she was also living. She has traveled the world twice over and has lived in the Midwest, Europe, Asia, and New York City. She froze her eggs in 2015.

Last, you will hear from **HEIDI,** thirty-seven. She runs a branding agency but is also highly involved in the nonprofit world. Heidi splits her time between New York and rural Pennsylvania, and is incredibly articulate; each thing she says is well considered and deeply informed. A fervent feminist, she has provocative things to say about how taking charge of our fertility is almost a radical act. And in at least one way, Heidi is different from the other women you have just met: after freezing her eggs a few years ago, she felt *less* sure that she even wanted to have children. Taking the time pressure off herself freed her up to think about what she genuinely wanted, and not just what she *thought* she wanted.

Let these women and me tell you: Once you suffer the rude awakening of infertility, your lifelong confidence in your fertility can quickly give way to a lengthy period of kicking yourself for not knowing sooner. Overconfidence in one's fertility is a very real problem. There are studies that prove most women have a much higher sense of certainty about their ability to reproduce than is actually backed up by statistics.

Now, please do not misunderstand. I am not suggesting that women should have babies younger or before they're ready to, nor am I suggesting that *every* twenty-something should go out and freeze her eggs. But we do have to talk about our fertility and reproductive health earlier and more proactively. We are proactive about cervical cancer—we get regular pap smears. We are proactive about breast cancer—we start getting mammograms at forty.

We do all kinds of things to ensure the future we want—plan for retirement, mind our credit scores, climb the corporate ladder, sock away savings. So why is there not a simple blood test offered up in our twenties to understand at least the direction of our reproductive potential, given that it will affect our futures tremendously, and given that there *are* steps we can take to maximize our chances of becoming mothers if we so desire?

I admit that had I known when I was in my twenties that getting pregnant might be difficult for me, it is doubtful I would have done anything drastically different. I would not have tried to have babies in my twenties. Egg freezing would not have been a financially viable option for me then (nor would it have been accessible, as it was labeled an experimental treatment until just recently), so I would not have run out to do that either. But I might have begun saving for the expensive eventuality of fertility treatments. I might have adopted a different mind-set, a more realistic approach, leaving me less shocked and frustrated when I hit a roadblock. In short, I might have gone into infertility prepared, instead of letting it blindside me.

Nearly five years after first attempting to get pregnant, I still do not know how the story ends for me. I am past my prime baby-making years, and paying for fertility treatments on one salary might lead me straight into bankruptcy rather than motherhood (or maybe both, making me a broke single mom—great!). But if I never end up having babies, I want to at least pass this lesson on to anyone who will listen, and to start driving earlier conversations about this topic.

My goal is not to scare you or encourage you to drop everything and get pregnant this second. Quite the opposite, actually. I'm simply acknowledging that baby making is happening later and later in life, which is fine, but, as such, my aim is to make you aware, and make the subject of egg freezing and fertility treatments—hell, fertility in general—perfectly normal and highly accessible. My hope is that heightened dialogue about this topic will eventually drive demand and, as a result, that fertility treatments will simply become part of our standard reproductive healthcare options.

I will try and make this easy and fast reading, so you can get back to the party, to saving the world, to working hard at building your career—in short, to whatever it is you would rather be doing than talking about your reproductive potential.

First off, a little tough love:

CAN YOU HANDLE THE TRUTH?

Ladies, I will not lie—this book is not for everyone. It is a reality check. If you are a tender soul who prefers not to face facts, set this book down now, because it is not for you. But if any of the following happens to be true for you, keep right on reading!

1. You have a vagina (literally and figuratively)

Facing facts requires the balls . . . wait, let me stop myself. Contrary to popular idiom, balls do not symbolize all that is gutsy. In fact, let's take a cue from Betty White, who once said, "Why do people say 'grow some balls'? Balls are weak and sensitive. If you wanna be tough, grow a vagina. Those things can take a pounding."

She is right. Women are tough. We have to be. Being a woman requires courage, strength, perseverance. Our feminist sisters of the past paved the way—so effectively, in fact, that we are now playing the same game as men. (The rules are often different for each sex, but that is another story.) And as you know, that is not always easy.

So let me rephrase: Reading this book requires a vagina. Literally, of course, but also figuratively. You need to be able to confront a few tough truths and figure out how to deal with them. It is time to face some facts that you may have ignored, denied, or tried to reason away. We *do* have a biological clock, and it *is* ticking, and time *does* run out. This is just the way it is—and it is time to realize that.

2. *You want all the information*

Victoria, one of the lovely ladies you just met, once told me that the greatest manifestation of success is having options in life. But having options requires knowing all the information. You need all the facts, even the inconvenient ones. If options require knowledge, and knowledge is power—well, you do the math.

You may not know if you want babies yet. But should you decide when you are, say, forty that you do want babies, I think you will agree that it would be nice to go into that decision educated, aware, and with options. Options like money you have saved for fertility treatments, or eggs you froze. Of course, you cannot have these options if you do not know they exist. Which is where I—and this book—come in.

Before we go any further, I want to acknowledge that fertility problems are not a reality for everyone. Turning thirty or thirty-five or even forty does not mean we are suddenly barren. Some lucky women are able to have babies naturally in their mid-forties. While I have a lot of friends who had serious fertility issues after a certain age, I also have some friends—not as many, I admit—who found themselves "accidentally" pregnant in their late thirties, or who really did not have to give it a second thought, and got pregnant easily. What I mean to say is that experiences vary, but you cannot simply hope to be in the minority of women who get pregnant later in life with very little difficulty.

This definitely should not sound like a lecture. Instead, I want this book to alert you to various information you may not have considered or simply did not know—because this information may very well influence one of the biggest decisions in your life.

So please read on—and be sure to bring your vagina with you.

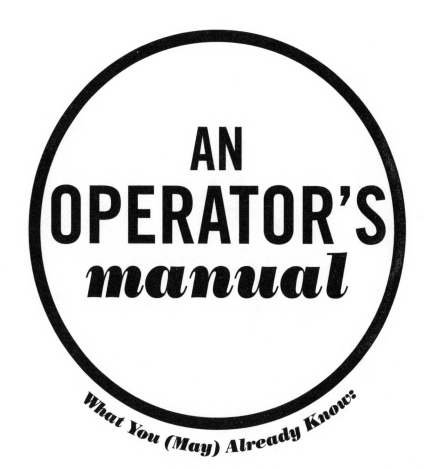

AN
OPERATOR'S
manual

What You (May) Already Know:

THE BASICS OF YOUR LADY BITS

A little female reproductive system Anatomy 101 is in order before we go any further, because all this fertility and egg-freezing talk makes a lot more sense if you know how a woman's body functions.

Sadly, many of us seem to know very little about our bodies—specifically our reproductive system, which is, by any metric, a pretty astonishing marvel of engineering. Most of us have only scratched the surface of what it does and how it works. Or, as Alison says, "I think it was around thirtyish, thirty-one maybe, when the question of fertility started to pop into my head. I was kind of just starting to think, *I wonder what I can find out about my fertility*. And as you may know, there is pretty close to nothing out there—few OBGYNs talk about it in the annual checkup, few fertility centers are doing any type of educational social campaigns around the power of knowledge. By the time I was thirty, I knew pretty much nothing at all about my own fertility. So being the proactive person I am, I just went into my OBGYN for a typical annual and said, 'Hey, I'm thirty-one and I'm worried about my fertility. I really want to have children someday. Is there anything I can find out now?' It was surprising to me that they really had never initiated that conversation, that I had to be the one to bring it up."

I could not agree more. So here is what most women *think* they know:

1. Women should get their periods once a month.
2. If a woman *does not* get her period once a month, it is because she is pregnant, has an eating disorder, is some kind of training-obsessed professional athlete or is on a form of birth control that interferes with her menstrual cycle. (Of course, there are other reasons women don't menstruate, like innate hormonal disorders

that affect ovulation, but I would argue that the average woman isn't even aware of this condition.)

I may be exaggerating a little—for example, some women may know that we also ovulate, and some women may know that it's nearly impossible to get pregnant while you're on your period. But essentially, our knowledge of what happens with our lady bits comes simply from what we can see on our panties once a month, not from an understanding of what's happening every month, inside our bodies. We have a clearer understanding of how our iPhones work than we do our own reproductive system. Unlike our iPhones, however, our bodies do not come with an operator's manual (or a Genius Bar to visit when they malfunction). So I am going to try to provide you with one. Here goes:

Let's call our reproductive body parts the *hardware*. First item in our hardware inventory: the vagina. I know you know what it is, but let's be clear about the purposes it serves. First, it is the site of sexual intercourse, and therefore serves as the highway for baby batter. It is also the conduit through which we release our menstrual blood and—one day, maybe—a baby. Honestly, that is sort of it. (Well, *functionally* speaking that is about it—though as anyone who has spent any time down there knows, the vagina has lots of other, more recreational uses.)

Next up is the cervix, the barrier between the vagina and the uterus. The cervix produces cervical mucus (gross), which can help promote conception. When you ovulate each month, you likely find that gooey stuff on your undies (also gross—and annoying). That goo is cervical mucus, and it is meant to help the sperm meet the egg. Think of the cervix as a Slip 'N Slide, and the cervical mucus as the sprinkler's helpful water; that slick substance—which is much thicker and less penetrable during the rest of the menstrual cycle—acts as a sperm reservoir, allowing sperm to slowly release and propel themselves through the cervix into your uterus.

Speaking of which, the uterus is a kind of embryonic studio apartment: it houses the embryo, or fertilized egg, and will be the baby's home until birth; we also refer to it as the womb. The uterus is amazingly flexible. Under normal conditions, it is about the size and shape of a pear, but it can, lest we forget, expand to accommodate a whole infant. It is also a super-strong organ (I told you, our lady bits are impressive!), able to contract forcefully enough during labor to shoot a baby out into the world.

Our fallopian tubes (also known as oviducts or uterine tubes) are the little passages through which eggs are transported to the uterus from the ovary each month. When an egg is fertilized, the tubes transport it to the uterus for implantation. (Perhaps you have heard someone say she has had her "tubes tied," once she is finished having children? These would be the tubes she is talking about.)

Now for the all-important ovary. Most everyone is born with two of them, and like all good team players (or those rare roommates who actually get along and each pull their weight), ovaries take turns. Each month, one ovary grows and releases an egg, from menarche (your first period) to menopause. The ovaries serve two purposes. One is to release an egg every month, and the other is to produce hormones—estrogen, progesterone, and testosterone. (Not to worry, you will be reading *lots* more about those hormones later on.)

Finally, there is the pituitary gland. While not technically in your reproductive region—in fact, it is located at the base of the brain—the pituitary is an incredibly important piece of your reproductive hardware. It releases two essential hormones related to the menstrual cycle, luteinizing hormone (LH) and follicle-stimulating hormone (FSH). (You will read more about those too.) Without these hormones, eggs do not develop, and ovulation (the release of a developed egg) does not occur. Thus, there is no potential for pregnancy.

Next, let's talk about the menstrual cycle—we will call that the *operating system*. The menstrual cycle involves a whole lot more than the few days of the month that we have our periods (or the week prior, when everything is sad and everyone is irritating). Think of it as the operating platform on which our reproductive system functions—the iOS installed on our anatomical hardware. Without it, that hardware is, in baby-making terms, pretty much useless.

Simply put, the menstrual cycle is governed by hormonal shifts that trigger changes in the ovaries and the lining of the uterus. It usually lasts about a month (in most women, it ranges from twenty-eight to thirty-five days). The cycle involves the preparation of an egg for fertilization, and ends with either a period or a pregnancy. (If it is the former, you go buy tampons; if it is the latter, you go lie down and think about how your entire life is about to change.)

The menstrual cycle is made up of four phases:

1. MENSTRUATION: Yeah, this one is pretty obvious to anyone older than twelve. It is the process by which your body sheds the soft tissue and blood vessels that make up the uterine lining—if no one (hint, hint: an embryo) is living in there, there is no need to keep the home furnished! It looks like a lot of blood. (Okay, sometimes it *is* a lot of blood.) This bleeding happens because estrogen and progesterone levels decrease after being ramped up during your last menstrual cycle.

2. FOLLICULAR: This stage starts at the same time as menstruation (when you begin to bleed), but it focuses on the development of ovarian follicles, the many sacs within the ovary that each contain a single egg. The follicles know to grow and develop because one of the hormones from the pituitary gland—follicle-stimulating hormone—increases at this time. A small group of growing follicles competes for dominance, but usually only one rises above the fray to become the candidate for fertilization. The dominant follicle makes estrogen, which tells the uterus to start getting ready for the egg's arrival and also, along with follicle size, causes a surge-release of luteinizing hormone, the ovulation trigger.

3. OVULATORY: This phase begins when luteinizing hormone surges and ends when it causes the dominant ovarian follicle to burst and release a mature egg. The egg then travels to the fallopian tube, where it dies a pretty quick death unless it meets up with one lucky sperm (eggs have about twelve to twenty-four hours to get themselves fertilized). You can get pregnant without actually having sex timed exactly to ovulation because sperm can survive inside the female reproductive hardware for several days, "waiting" for the egg to become available. The fact remains: the twenty-four *hours* after the egg is released is the only time of our cycle when we can get pregnant.

4. LUTEAL: After ovulation has occurred, luteinizing hormone and follicle-stimulating hormone levels decrease. In addition, the ruptured follicle that released the egg magically transforms into what is known as the corpus luteum, or a factory that produces the hormone progesterone. Along with estrogen, progesterone prepares the lining of the uterus, in hopes of making it a cozy nine-month crash pad for a fertilized egg. If you get knocked up, the cells around the growing embryo begin to make the pregnancy hormone, human chorionic gonadotropin (hCG)—the one that causes a urine pregnancy test to be positive. When present, this hormone maintains the corpus luteum for an additional two months, producing the progesterone necessary to maintain a growing fetus until it can manufacture its own hormones. However, if your egg is not fertilized, the corpus luteum shuts down the factory and stops making progesterone, and estrogen also decreases. These abrupt hormonal changes signal to your body that it's time to start menstruation. And then you start all over again! Fun, right?

Now that we have the hardware and the operating system down, let's dig into the *software*, or the hormones that regulate our menstrual cycle. When we hear the word "hormones," most of us probably think of moody teenagers or PMS-stricken (or menopausal) women. But they are more than just the triggers for vicious mood swings and hot flashes. Hormones also regulate when we release our eggs, and serve a tremendous role in determining if we conceive and, when we do, whether we carry a healthy pregnancy to term. There are many different hormones that course through our bodies, but because this is not a textbook and you have things to do, we will just cover those that relate to our cycle and fertility.

To simplify, let's divide hormones into two groups. In the first group are the hormones largely made by our sex organs: estrogen and progesterone. In the second group, the "smart" hormones made by the brain, which are the aforementioned follicle-stimulating hormone (FSH) and luteinizing hormone (LH). (Okay, these last two are not actually *smarter*, per se, but they do come from the brain.)

The hormones in the first group, estrogen and progesterone, are, simply put, the hormones that both give us our female characteristics and make pregnancy possible. Estrogen is a female steroid hormone mainly produced by the ovaries. It's responsible for endowing us with breasts, wider hips, and higher fat levels—like I said, the things that make us look like women. Estrogen levels rise and fall over the course of our cycles, with levels peaking at the end of the follicular phase, right before ovulation. These high levels thicken the endometrium, making the uterus a suitable home for an embryo, just in case fertilization happens to occur in that twenty-four-hour window after ovulation. Estrogen is also an important player outside of your lady parts, acting on the bones, brain, and many other organs. This is all to say that it's an important hormone for women to keep in check.

Progesterone is the hormone that helps with final preparation and maintenance of the lining of the uterus to receive and nourish a future baby during the luteal phase. If no future baby comes knocking, progesterone and estrogen levels drop, the uterine lining breaks down, and menstruation occurs. If pregnancy occurs, the placenta (the embryo's source of nutrition), produces mass quantities of progesterone throughout the remaining pregnancy. Along with estrogen, this progesterone stops you from releasing more eggs once you are already knocked up.

The hormones released from the pituitary gland include FSH and LH. FSH stimulates egg maturation and follicle growth. FSH levels are one of the things doctors measure to assess your ovarian reserve (translation: how many eggs you have left and the quality of the ones that remain). It is typically measured on day two or three of your menstrual cycle. LH is only released from the pituitary when a certain amount of estrogen has been produced and the follicle matures and is ready to release the egg. About thirty-six hours after the LH surge, the follicle breaks, releasing the egg from the ovary. LH is what ovulation kits test for, because a high presence of LH signals the onset of ovulation (actually, the time just *before* ovulation, which, if you are trying to get pregnant, is exactly the moment you should start having a lot of sex). LH also converts the broken follicle into a corpus luteum, that progesterone-making factory that prepares the endometrium for the potential arrival of a fertilized egg.

Finally, a curveball: there is actually one more hormone you should know about, which is anti-Mullerian hormone (AMH). It's a hormone produced by granulosa cells of the ovary during the reproductive years. AMH is one of the best indicators of ovarian reserve, so it is an important hormone to keep in mind as we get into all the fun fertility stuff to come.

Which is exactly where we are heading now that we have all that boring (but important!) stuff out of the way. Next, let's move on to what they do not teach you in sex education (but really, really should).

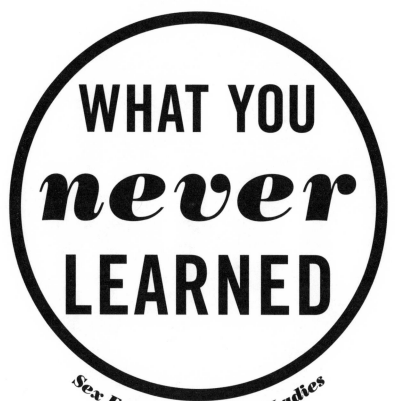

WHAT YOU *never* LEARNED

Sex Ed Let You Down, Ladies

There is sex education, and then there is what I call *higher* sex education. If the former only taught us about prevention—and the total life ruination, after-school-special style, of accidental pregnancy—the latter aims to broaden our reproductive understanding and help us take proactive control of it. As I said, we often obtain this higher form of sex education only after we have been actively trying to conceive but are finding ourselves unable to do so. That is a real shame, and it is exactly what I hope to remedy in the pages to come.

Sex education—taught in junior high or high school, with its strange slideshows and awkward references to wet dreams—has inarguably encouraged and assisted the upward trajectory of modern women, encouraging them to exercise agency in their sexual lives and to be informed about their bodies, and the damage that having babies prematurely can do. It has also, to be perfectly frank, really let us down.

But let me back up for a moment and give credit where credit is due. The upside of sex education is obvious. It serves as a necessary acknowledgment that teenagers are horny, curious little beings who, more likely than not, will experiment with sex. And because sex comes with consequences—especially when we are young, naive, and fertile—it is of course tremendously important that we be apprised of all the facts. The universal implementation of sex education in the 1980s and '90s was controversial, but it ultimately helped curb the AIDS and teen pregnancy epidemics that had been rampant in this country before that. In fact, according to the Guttmacher Institute, US teen pregnancy, birth, and abortion rates have declined by as much as 51 percent since their high point in the 1990s. Sex ed bears a lot of responsibility for that happy shift.

And while the percentages vary by state and demographic, that decline continues to this day. Sex ed has sparked a significant shift in how our culture views young parents—in fact, can you even *think* of a peer who had a baby before she was eighteen? Probably not. What would have been no big deal at all in your mom's or grandmother's generations—when young women routinely became pregnant before their twenty-fifth birthday—has become, if not taboo, at the very least a serious rarity in most parts of the country. Similarly, the rate of contraction of AIDS and HIV are also on a sharp decline, falling by one-third in the past decade alone.

So what beef could I possibly have with sex education, you ask? I believe sex education also fostered a lot of ignorance, because what we learned in high school simply was not the whole truth, but it was presented to us as though it was. That is dangerous. The resulting gaps in our knowledge were, for most of us, never filled in. In my experience, sex education only taught us about the *don'ts*, about the things to avoid—namely, pregnancy and STDs. And of course, there is merit in that. Teens need to know how to protect themselves. But unlike the subject of, say, American history, which is typically elaborated upon at length when we get to college, our understanding of our reproductive system never seems to be readdressed once we become proper adults (unless you're studying human biology, of course, but it is not addressed in any general curriculum). At least not until that ill-understood reproductive system up and fails us.

Now let's address a few of the gaps in our knowledge:

1. It is not as easy to get pregnant as you may think.

I went through high school, college, and all of my twenties trying *not* to get knocked up. I cannot even count how many "scares" I had—buying the little plastic sticks at the drugstore, urgently waiting for that line in the little window to pop up. Of course, it was probably good that I was so focused on prevention—because God knows that I, pregnant in my twenties, would most definitely have been a disaster. But I was mistaken in taking for granted that I could get pregnant at any given moment.

You might be feeling exactly the same way. Many of my friends made the same assumption when they were younger. As Ana says, "In my twenties, I thought about my fertility in that I assumed that I *was* fertile and could just get pregnant any time. I didn't really think about it being a problem."

During my marriage, I finally got a glimpse of how difficult getting pregnant can be. I was healthy. I was relatively young—in my early thirties. There was no identifiable reason for my infertility. And yet I still had trouble getting knocked up. I soon learned that being in my thirties alone could be a reason for my infertility. (What? I had never known this. Forties, I could understand, but thirties?) This was also when I found out that getting pregnant is not even a tenth as simple as I had been led to believe for all those naive, youthful years. I remember thinking, *Why the hell didn't anyone tell me this?*

Even if you have sex every day, you are not meaningfully changing the odds, especially as you age, considering that you can only get pregnant a few days out of the month. And even if you do have sex on those fertile days, there is still no guarantee that you will get pregnant. Dr. Noyes usually tells her patients that fecundity (or reproductive rate) is about 20 percent per cycle (and if nothing is wrong, most young people will get pregnant within five months of trying). Healthy women between the ages of nineteen and twenty-six have about a 50 percent chance of getting pregnant even *on their most fertile days*. On average, women aged twenty-seven to thirty-four have less than a 40 percent chance of conceiving *on their most fertile days*. And women thirty-five to thirty-nine have less than a 30 percent chance of getting pregnant *on their most fertile days*.

My youthful caution, while well intended, was clearly based on far too little information. I assumed, as sex ed had *led* me to assume, that I could get pregnant at any time. I never questioned that assumption. I mean, look at birth control pills: There is a pill in that pack for every single day of the month, right? Which implied, at least to my mind, that every day is a potentially fertile one. I never questioned that assumption, either.

What I did not realize, and what so many women do not realize, is that there is a lot more to getting pregnant than just having sex without protection. Our eggs are not just hanging out, waiting for Mr. Right to come along. Our eggs show up once a month, and that appearance is, as they say in show business, a limited engagement. The window for potential fertilization is extremely small. And even if an egg turns up and is ready to go at just the right time, the sperm may not make their date. Our vagina's environment kills or traps most of them, and still others simply cannot make it through the mucus filled challenge course of our lady bits to where our egg awaits to be fertilized. Only the very determined little swimmers make it.

But okay, let's say a few good swimmers make it up there. They have to be resolute and unwavering in their efforts to burrow through the wall of the egg. (We have all seen *Look Who's Talking*, right? Or maybe you are too young for that reference?) And *if* that happens, and your monthly egg is lucky enough to be fertilized by the Michael Phelps of sperm, you still have to hope for implantation in the uterine wall (the little embryo needs to burrow right in there like a tick) and, beyond that, a successful first trimester (according to Dr. Sarah Druckenmiller of NYU Langone Medical Center, approximately one-third of all pregnancies end in miscarriage).

That is one hell of a well-timed, precise process! And here we thought it was easy.

Kate knows firsthand just how difficult it can be to get pregnant. "I thought I had plenty of time," she says. "I think I did what a lot of women who are successful do: I ran my own life, did my own thing. I didn't have any qualms that motherhood would happen for me. I wasn't overly worried. I suspected, having been a high achiever all my life, that I was going to get an A or B grade in this too." Of course, that was not the case.

Now, I realize that lots of people get pregnant accidentally. In fact, I have friends who could not help but get knocked up once a year in their twenties! But once you know what a pregnancy involves, the word "accident" starts to sound like a misnomer. Pregnancies are the result of a series of carefully orchestrated events, of everything working together at just the right moment. A lot has to happen, with impeccable timing, for you to get pregnant. And that is something you need to know.

2. There are things about the pill you probably have not considered.

We have been on the pill for a long time—nearly sixty years, in fact. In 1960 the FDA officially approved the pill for contraceptive use, and you will not be at all surprised to hear that it was an instant hit. We ladies were popping them like candy: By 1963 more than two million American women were on the pill. Now, this being a women's rights issue, female contraception was not without controversy. Religious leaders and conservatives of the day were outraged. After all, the pill formally recognized a woman's desire to have recreational sex—that is, sex with men to whom we might not be married, or, if we *were* married, sex without the sacred aim of motherhood. Scandal!

This monumental change was incredibly important for womankind and was, I would argue, inextricably linked to the second-wave feminist movement. The 1960s were a historic, milestone decade for women. Not only was Title VII of the 1964 Civil Rights Act passed (prohibiting employment discrimination on the basis of sex, race, and religion), a cultural movement began to bubble up—a movement that questioned the "all-American family" facade. Having children and keeping house need not be a woman's entire reason for living, it said.

Betty Friedan's bombshell book *The Feminine Mystique*, published in 1963, revealed that while many American women were living in relative comfort—complete with husband, kids, white picket fence, the whole pretty picture—secretly, they suffered significant unhappiness. It turns out that only having the option to be a homemaker was not as satisfying as women of that generation had been led to believe (shocking, I know). The book was an instant bestseller, inspiring hundreds of thousands of women to seek fulfillment outside the home.

What does all this have to do with the pill? Well, much of this upward trajectory I have just described would not have been possible without it. If women simply continued to have babies with no real say in when—or whether—they wanted to conceive, their ability to step boldly into the world and find their passions and careers, to create the lives they wanted to live, would have been greatly diminished. The pill means options. Options, as I said earlier, mean freedom.

But I do think we should be more aware of what we are doing when we take oral birth control—or any daily medication, for that matter. Many women today take the pill for granted, swallowing it down for years at a time without much thought. The pill brings with it some rare but serious potential dangers, such as an increased risk of blood clots and heart disease. It can also raise your blood pressure. The pill has also been associated with an increased risk of certain cancers, such as those of the cervix and central nervous system.

I am not saying we should all get off the pill. But ladies, the time of our peak fertility, when it is near effortless for most of us to get pregnant, is limited. So let's at least *consider* the ramifications before signing up for years of a daily dose of estrogen. Take the pill if it is right for you, but do not take it blindly.

3. Birth control is not actually control; it is simply prevention.

My Birth Control 2.0 idea is all about expanding the conversation around birth control to include more than just not getting pregnant.

Let's talk about how to be proactive about our reproductive futures through simple blood tests that offer a general indication of our fertility and, potentially, egg freezing. Let's help women make their own decisions based on facts and statistics. Even if you finish this book believing everything I have said is absurd—that these are indeed the rantings of a crazy woman, and that freezing your eggs is little more than an efficient means of throwing thousands of dollars away—at least take with you the idea that you deserve to make decisions about your fertility future that are based in fact. Which, of course, means finding out those facts.

Let's talk semantics for a moment, because words do matter— they inform paradigms and ways of thinking. "Birth control," as defined by Oxford dictionaries is "the practice of preventing unwanted pregnancies, typically by use of contraception." By contrast, the definition of "control" is "the power to influence or direct people's behavior or course of events."

So the definition of "control" changes when it is in the context of "birth control." It comes to mean prevention—not proactive decision making. The true meaning of "control" is much broader on its own and, I would argue, needs to be much broader when applied to birth control. Who cares, you ask? We should. Because this narrow definition of birth control results in only one conversation: how not to get pregnant. It leaves no room for taking charge of your fertility, or for talking about reproductive health in general.

Now that we are all well versed in not getting pregnant, let's look at the full spectrum of birth control, from prevention to the decisive effort to have a baby. In other words, let's adopt this Birth Control 2.0 idea (and not just because I coined it). The way we think about birth control has not evolved since its inception—it has always been about prevention. It is time to broaden that definition, especially as our societal "problem" swings from too many unwanted pregnancies among young women to too many women finding themselves infertile and trying to have a baby later in life.

4. *Your gynecologist is more than just a pill-pusher.*

I once asked Laura—my friend who is a lesbian—how she thinks she will have a baby one day. "Will you carry? Will your future partner carry? Will you adopt? Will you use a surrogate?" I pelted her with questions until finally she looked at me like I had five heads and said, "Agnes, before you started your blog, I had zero idea about my reproductive system or how it all works, so I have no idea yet how I will have a baby. I'm still getting over the fact that I ovulate." As a lesbian, she had never had to worry about birth control and, as a result, had never really thought about her reproductive system or her fertility. That says a lot about how little some in the gynecological profession tell us about our bodies, and, as a result, how many of us come to see those doctors largely as birth control dispensaries. Even worse, many women simply do not visit the gynecologist on a regular basis, despite recommendations that they undergo a basic checkup every year.

Laura went on to tell me that she did not see a gynecologist for the first time until she was around thirty, because she views them as doctors who simply dole out birth control pills. As a woman who only has sex with other women, she felt that a gyno was totally unnecessary for her. Now, this is obviously an extreme case, but it does emphasize that most of us are only having one conversation with our gynecologists, and it centers on avoiding pregnancy.

Shockingly, the average woman only spends about twelve minutes per year talking to her gynecologist. That is obviously not a lot of time to discuss future pregnancy or fertility so it's no wonder so many women never discuss it proactively. Let's break it down:

HOW WE CHEAT OURSELVES AT THE DOCTOR'S OFFICE
(If We Go At All)

45% of women who have never had an abnormal pap smear do not see a gynecologist annually

52% percent of women between the ages of twenty-five and thirty-five have never discussed future pregnancy plans with their gynecologists

78% have never discussed age as a factor in pregnancy

89–96% of women between the ages of twenty-five and thirty-five never talk about fertility treatments

Research has shown that women believe it is far easier to get pregnant than it is, and they underestimate the amount of time it takes and the effect of their age on their fertility. In fact, nine out of ten women gravely underestimated the rate of infertility problems among women forty and older.

If none of this inspires you to start having a different dialogue with your doctor, consider this: The "head in the sand" approach will only cost *you*. There is no other aspect of our health and well-being that we leave to chance as much as our ability to start a family—which is stunning when you consider the emotional relationship women have with becoming mothers. Somehow it seems there is an inverse correlation between how much we care about motherhood and how much we are willing to do to increase our chances of achieving it. We drink milk as children to make sure we grow healthy bones, exercise to keep our hearts strong and our arteries unclogged, brush our teeth twice daily to prevent cavities, yet we do nothing to protect our fertility.

What to do about this? Start asking questions! (More on that later.)

In addition to asking questions, ask to have tests done to determine your FSH and AMH levels. Measuring these levels allows a doctor to assess your ovarian reserve, and how hard your body has to work to create follicles. A high FSH number is not a good sign; in fact, when women approach menopause, their FSH levels increase greatly because their body is still trying to produce follicles (persistent little things, aren't they?). As I mentioned, you should also ask to have your AMH levels tested. As you learned earlier, AMH is the anti-mullerian hormone, and is another good indicator of your ovarian reserve. Unlike with FSH, you want these numbers to be higher. Here is a breakdown:

INTERPRETATION (women younger than age 35)	AMH Blood Level
High (often PCOS)	Over 4.0 ng/ml
Normal	1.5–4.0 ng/ml
Low Normal Range	1.0–1.5 ng/ml
Low	0.5–1.0 ng/ml
Very Low	Less than 0.5 ng/ml

This information is well worth knowing, because it fosters a dialogue between you and your gynecologist—and you need a doctor who is willing to be a partner in your fertility journey.

Kate gets fired up when it comes to this subject. "This is one of the things that pisses me off," she says. "Why isn't this information about infertility associated with age more widely discussed—even by the relevant doctors? Why didn't my OBGYN tell me that my fertility was a factor when I was considering my life and how to struc-ture it? The timelines stretch out massively; you don't just wake up one morning and say *I think I'll do IVF*, and then do it the next day. A lot of women begin at the point where they really should be stop-ping, because nobody has had the conversation with them in their twenties. That's a bugbear, and the medical profession is really taking its time catching up."

5. You do have a biological clock (and it is ticking).

I used to think that only men—especially men in cities like New York and Los Angeles, where gorgeous women abound—suffered from Peter Pan syndrome. But ladies, I have since realized that we suffer from it as well.

In my survey of hundreds of women across the country, I have found that, as it relates to having babies, we have embraced a form of magical thinking. We deny our biological clock, telling ourselves we have more time than we do. Now, with all due respect to men, this female form of Peter Pan syndrome is not as douchey as the male strain (theirs is more about refusing to grow up, while ours is about refusing to acknowledge that we already have), but it does exist. Simply put, we are having fun, concentrating on careers and financial independence, in denial about the fact that we simply do not have all the time in the world. In fact, in conducting my survey, I came to a startling conclusion: the older the woman, the more time she thinks she has to get pregnant. That was a troubling finding, to say the least.

So listen up, Tinker Bell. This is not Never Never Land. You will, in fact, age. So will your ovaries, and every little egg inside them. While you may not want to have a baby this instant—which is perfectly fine—you should at least acknowledge that the biologi-cal clock is not some antiquated notion meant to induce panic and convince us to settle down early.

Remember when I cited some statistics that say our chances of pregnancy decline significantly as we age, and that our eggs age right along with us? Here are a few nuggets of information to drive the point home:

THE HARD-BOILED FACTS ON EGGS

Egg donors are typically required to be younger than thirty years of age. Why do you think other people do not want your eggs after thirty? Because young eggs are better than old eggs. Period.

The number of eggs present in a woman's ovaries actually peaks while she is still in the womb, where she is carrying around six or seven million eggs. And it is all downhill from there! In fact, by the time we are born, we are left with only one or two million. And by the time we hit puberty and start our periods, we are left with just a few hundred thousand. Of course, not all of those will mature and become viable. In fact, most will not.

For an average, healthy woman, the decline in fertility potential starts in her early thirties and significantly accelerates during her mid to late thirties. According to Dr. Noyes, women can lose up to $2/3$ of their fertility potential between the ages of 35 and 40, with the decline rate at about 15% per year over that critical 5-year time period.

This decline in fertility is not just due to the dwindling number of eggs, it is also because we're left with fewer "good" eggs, or eggs that are healthy enough to be fertilized. So while we may technically be ovulating, the eggs we are dropping are less likely to result in a healthy baby.

In fact, the genetic material inside the egg starts to mutate around the age of thirty-five—which is why pregnant women older than that are typically advised to undergo more serious genetic tests.

We spend so much time thinking about and fretting over how our outsides change with time—expensive eye creams and other forms of hope in a jar, not to mention neck lifts and Botox, make up a large part of the "aging" conversation. But you would not be wrong to think about your insides the same way. Wrinkly skin and saggy breasts are not the only things that show our age. Our ovaries and their contents do too. Think of the changes they undergo as similar to getting crow's-feet or drooping eyelids, or losing skin elasticity—just with more significant medical consequences.

6. Guys have a biological clock, too.

Many of us know at least one older man—you know, *that* older man, the one with the hot young wife and a little brood of babies conceived with said hot young wife. Michael Douglas and Catherine Zeta Jones had their second child when he was fifty-eight and she was thirty-three. Rod Stewart famously had a child at sixty-six; his oldest daughter had her first child around the same time, so he had a baby and a grandkid simultaneously. Though he has nothing on Mick Jagger, who happens to have a great-grandchild who is older than one of his children. (Eew.) The list of old celebrity dads is a long one: George Lucas (he was sixty-nine), Steve Martin (sixty-seven), Robert De Niro (sixty-eight). I could go on.

While it is far more common for older men to naturally produce babies than it is for older women to get pregnant, men also experience changes to their fertility as they age. We rarely think about a man's age as a potential barrier to having a child, and the studies I have found on the subject sometimes have conflicting information about how old is too old for a man, but the reality is that just like our eggs age and become less viable, so too does a man's baby batter. In fact, there comes an age when it ceases to be baby batter—after that, it is just batter.

A few notable facts on this subject:

THE SKINNY ON SPERM

While we commonly blame the age of a woman on a couple's inability to conceive (and conceive a healthy child), there is growing evidence that the age of a man contributes significantly as well, both in natural and assisted conception.

- According to the Avon Longitudinal Study of Pregnancy and Childhood, men older than 35 had a 50% lower chance of conceiving within 12 months than men 25 and under; this study was conducted among couples who ultimately had a baby, but it does suggest that it takes longer with older sperm.

- Several hormonal changes occur as men age—it's not just us ladies that deal with hormonal realities. I won't bore you with the specifics, but these hormonal changes lead to lower libido (I can confirm this from my own personal experiences with older gentlemen!), impaired erectile function (thank God for Viagra!), and poor semen quality.

- In a prospective study of 23,821 pregnant women followed in the Danish National Birth Cohort study, pregnancies initiated by men 50 or older had a twofold increased risk of ending in fetal loss.

- Some studies have shown that fathers older than 55 years had 4.4 times increased risk of having an offspring with autism (this is after controlling for things like maternal age and parental psychiatric history).

These facts are important to bear in mind, because the longer we wait to have kids, the older we will be, and thus, more than likely, the older our potential mates will be (unless you prefer a younger man, of course, and there's nothing wrong with that!). If you have always assumed that a man can get you pregnant well into his golden years, consider the health of the potential children born from his not-so-golden sperm. And if you decide to get pregnant through a donor, err on the side of young, strapping sperm. There are plenty of Mick Jaggers out there, but there are also a significant number of average Joes who will lose the ability to impregnate us with time.

7. *Fertility is solely a women's issue.*

Yes, men's biological clocks are a factor in the quest to get pregnant. But when it comes to the process of battling infertility, it is the woman who tends to carry the greatest burden, regardless of whether the problem is with the eggs or the sperm.

By the time my ex and I finally went to my doctor, it had been well over a year of us trying on our own. But when I say "on our own," what I really mean is on *my* own. Sure, he contributed the sperm, but beyond that, everything was my job. I was the one who had to pee on an ovulation test stick several days each month while hiding out in my office bathroom (the best time to test for ovulation is mid-morning—in other words, prime work hours). I was the one who researched clinics and doctors. And during our first consultation, our doctor made it perfectly clear that making a baby would continue to be my problem. She said we would both be tested for all kinds of potential barriers to conception (he for sperm count and motility, me for ovarian reserve and any anatomical anomalies), but no matter who had the problem, I would be the one getting routinely poked and prodded going forward.

The bizarre thing was that his sperm and reproductive health were more than healthy, and my ovarian reserve and reproductive organs were in tip-top shape. And so we had what doctors call "unidentified infertility" (to me this translates to: "You are either too old or too stressed."). And somehow, in the strange fog of injections and test sticks, doctor visits and crying jags, this failure became all about me. It wasn't that *we* could not get pregnant; it was that *I* could not get pregnant.

Let me make a little list to demonstrate how this works and why this is our problem, ladies:

LADIES

Pre-Fertility Treatment

Have conversation with gynecologist about fact that you are trying get pregnant.

Buy ovulation kits and then pee on stick after stick, usually at work.

Make time to have sex around the small window of ovulation, regardless of whether you are in the mood or whether it is convenient.

Continue this process of checking ovulation kits and having timed sex for three to twelve months, depending on your age. All the while, attempting to preserve sexiness of your sex so you and your partner do not begin to view it as chore.

Fertility Treatment, Part 1

Research best doctors and clinics, whether or not said doctors and clinics take insurance, and whether or not said insurance even covers fertility treatments; wince at thought of paying out of pocket.

Make appointment months in advance, and make sure partner is available for initial consultation.

Undergo non-invasive tests (blood work, etc.).

Undergo more invasive tests (vaginal ultrasounds, etc.) to determine follicle counts; undergo even more invasive hysterosalpingogram test to determine whether or not there are any blockages in uterus and fallopian tubes.

Fertility Treatment, Part 2

Depending on test results, start course of oral drugs (Clomid, letrozole, etc.).

Continue to time sex based on ovulation (all while still trying to keep it sexy).

Fertility Treatment, Part 2 (continued)

Anxiously await time of month when you should have your period, bracing for worst; stop drinking alcohol, and coffee in case you are finally pregnant.

Fertility Treatment, Part 3

Start injections to stimulate follicle production.

Have (incredibly uncomfortable) catheter inserted into uterus where washed sperm are released closer to site where fertilization can take place.

Fertility Treatment, Part 4

If timed sex with Clomid or letrozole and IUI have failed, fun really starts: Begin daily injection of heavy-duty follicle-inducing hormones to increase the number of eggs matured and released from the ovaries, and time that with IUI—or, if proceding straight to IVF, take and even bigger dose of FSH to ensure production of as many healthy follicles possible.

Come into doctor's office several times a week to have follicle growth checked.

For IVF, when follicles mature, undergo minor surgery to remove eggs, which are fertilized by partner's sperm in a dish.

Continue with injections to make sure the uterus lining is optimally developed for embryo implantation; the fertilized egg is then placed in your body through the cervix.

Possibly repeat several times before it finally works.

Sometimes, rather than placing the embryo into the body in the same cycle as it is created, the embryo is instead tested for chromosomes and placed in the freezer, being used to try to create pregnancy in a subsequent month, a treatment cycle that requires more hormone usage.

GENTLEMEN

 ## Pre-Fertility Treatment

Ejaculate inside girlfriend/wife.

Fertility Treatment, Part 1

Join girlfriend/wife for consultation with doctor; nod along while scrolling through iPhone.

Maybe undergo some blood work.

Ejaculate into a cup.

Maybe take oral supplements or drugs.

Fertility Treatment, Part 2

Ejaculate inside girlfriend/wife.

Fertility Treatment, Part 3

Ejaculate into a cup again.

Fertility Treatment, Part 4

Ejaculate into a cup a few more times.

See what I mean? However supportive your mate may be, the overwhelming majority of the hard work of fertility treatments will fall to you, the woman.

But let's explore this idea from another angle. Fertility is a women's issue not only because the bulk of the treatment and research falls to you. It is also a women's issue because reproductive enlightenment is the ultimate form of feminism.

Let me explain. When it comes to being a woman in 2017, there is good news and there is bad news. I am going to start with the good news. Women are *rocking it* these days. Not only are we allowed to do whatever the boys do, we are *expected* to—and, more and more, we are allowed to do it while wearing a skirt and lipstick. We are slowly moving away from the days of having to conform to the corporate world by wearing awful pantsuits, squashing our femininity so we would be thought of as "serious" instead of frivolous. As my four-year-old niece likes to boast when we girls are hanging out getting mani-pedis, "We're girls!" Hell yeah, we're girls! My niece *loves* being a girl. She owns it. And hopefully, by the time she is an adult, nobody will ever hold her back for being a tutu-wearing, lipstick-loving, nail-polished girly girl. That is because the world is changing (albeit much slower than I would like). Increasingly, references to the business world's "boys club" are met with blank stares. Yes, there are still some stodgy old bastards out there who refuse to admit that women can be their equals—or superiors. Not to mention that you can still expect to earn less than your male counterparts, even if you are doing the same work. I am not saying that sexism has been eradicated. (It has not—oh, how it has not.) But what I *am* saying is that we have never had it better than this, ladies, and in my estimation, it is just going to get better and fairer from here.

Never before have we had such a deep influence on the world. In 2014, the most recent year for which such figures exist, nearly 60 percent of all master's degrees and 51 percent of doctorate degrees were earned by women. This critical mass of learned ladies is translating into real, societal shifts. In 2014, 22 percent of married households had female breadwinners (compared to 4 percent in 1970). Between 1997 and 2014, women-owned firms increased by nearly 70 percent! That's a rate of one and a half times more than the national average. That translates to increased revenues of 72 percent, exceeding the growth rates of all but the largest publicly traded firms—it tops growth rates of all other privately held businesses (so we're not talking about little arts and crafts businesses!). Our list of accomplishments goes on and on.

But cultural and societal evolution is not free—it brings with it a raft of larger implications, and we have largely ignored the ones that pertain to our fertility for far too long. While we no longer expect Prince Charming to spirit us off to our happy ending, we do wait for the right guy, refusing to settle for less. Which is great! Except . . . there is a clock on our fertility. We may have broken the glass ceiling, but we have not yet outsmarted nature.

This book is about pointing out a few elephants in the room—discussing the options we have to preserve our fertility, and our reproductive health in general. Doing so is an inherently feminist act. Once we know that time is limited, and once we have the necessary information about our bodies, our options, and our needs, we can take control of our reproductive journey, navigating our fates proactively.

Think of the lax way in which men conduct relationships: if they are not into it, they bail. Wouldn't it be fun to have the same attitude that so many of them do? If we know we are covered, fertility-wise, that becomes a real possibility. We can afford to hold out without worry. And we can accomplish even more, because during those crucial years, instead of making babies, we can spend our energy building our dreams, starting companies, writing books, making movies, going to Mars—in short, we can spend our twenties and thirties doing whatever the hell we want, just like men do.

While there are no guarantees, freezing your eggs—and otherwise knowing what is going on with your fertility—can take some of the pressure off. It can also give you the time and opportunity to decide if children are really what you want, and not just what you *think* you want. It may surprise you to hear this, but some women who freeze their eggs—who go through that considerable trouble and expense—ultimately come to realize they do not want children after all. Once they give themselves the option, they decide not to exercise it. It may seem counterintuitive, but it makes sense if you think about it. It is nearly impossible to make a rational, fully considered decision about anything that comes with a blaring ticking clock. Imagine if you were trying to order dinner at a restaurant, and as you deliberated between the hanger steak and the tilapia, the waiter politely explained that you had one second left to decide, or you would get nothing. Pretty much any one of us would blurt out an answer, hoping we had gone with what we actually wanted most. Remove the pressure, and you have time and space to actually think about whether beef would taste better than fish, or whether being a parent is definitely, positively, absolutely what you would prefer. Freezing your eggs lets you take the time to figure that out.

As I said earlier, Heidi had exactly this experience. She froze her eggs when she was thirty-four, which she felt was an important and necessary thing to do to take control of her fertility. All these years later, she is no longer all that sure she wants to be a mom. "Because I had that time, my opinion changed," she says. "I think there's this animal thing about becoming a mom, but I don't have it. Now that I've frozen my eggs, I look at my life, and I really *like* my life. And I don't really have a desire to have kids. If I met the right person and it was really important to him . . . I'm not one of those people saying 'Never, never, never.' But it's funny that now that I've spent—what? Twelve grand?—that *now* I realize I don't want to have kids. Kind of crazy."

The point is, it can be really hard to know what you actually want. And when I say "you," I mean *you*—not the culture you live in, not your family, not your future husband, and not some future version of you who finally has time to sort through all this fertility stuff. This is information you need now. And that is why this conversation is so important.

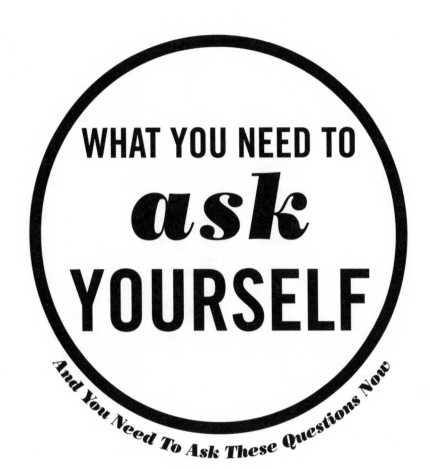

WHAT YOU NEED TO
ask
YOURSELF

And You Need To Ask These Questions Now

Before you map out what your own reproductive path will look like, it is important to ponder a few things you might not have considered. First, do you think you might ever want to be a mom (and more power to you if you do not!)? And if you think you do want to be a mom eventually, how do you picture it? Are you a young mom or an older mom? (In other words, when do you want to make this hypothetical baby happen?) If you begin to approach that cutoff age and find yourself without a male companion (or without a male companion eager to be a dad), will you consider doing the whole single-mom thing? And, before you go and start down the expensive path of egg freezing, do you consider the procedure to be an insurance policy—a little act of reassurance that makes you feel better that you will have options later in life—or do you see it more as an unproven gamble? And finally, if you start leaning toward egg freezing, examine why you are doing it. Go into it enlightened! And also know that the very act of freezing your eggs, of taking a bit of control, may enlighten you. You may decide, with a bit more time on your hands, that you do not need children to fulfill you as a woman, or make your life complete. Each of these questions is important, and let me be the one to tell you that you will be glad you asked them sooner rather than later.

1. How old is too old for me?

I have already talked a lot about how our eggs become less likely to result in a baby at a certain age—and how, sadly, that age may not be as far off as we would like to think. But let's pretend for a moment that the age of your eggs is a nonissue. If that is the case, the question becomes simpler: when will it feel right for you to become a mom?

The age of first-time mothers is currently on a steady incline, and has been for decades. However difficult it can be to get pregnant after your prime fertile years, older women *are* getting pregnant with their first babies more than ever before. But consider this: according to the Centers for Disease Control and Prevention, overall birth rates are in a steady decline in the United States, because women are waiting longer than ever. I am no social scientist, but to me the logic tracks: Because women are delaying pregnancy more than ever before, fewer of them are able to get pregnant once they are ready to. (Also, when we start later, we have fewer children.) The numbers do not lie—more women are having babies later:

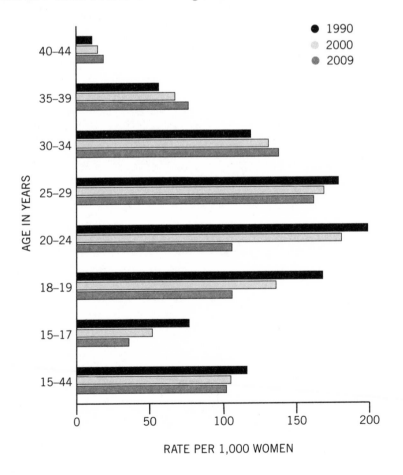

RATE PER 1,000 WOMEN

While this chart stops at age forty-four, there is actually a growing trend of women in their fifties and sixties giving birth. Yes, you read that correctly. Giving birth in your fifties may sound a little outrageous, but thanks to advancements in reproductive assistance, it is happening. As of this writing, the oldest recorded mother on Earth gave birth in India at the shocking age of seventy, to two-pound twins, via emergency cesarean section. (Note: she did not, of course, accomplish this with her own eggs.) In 2006, a woman set the record in the United States for oldest birth at the age of sixty.

While I truly believe every woman should have the right to have a baby at whatever age she sees fit—provided she can care for that baby—doing so in one's sixties or seventies is, to my mind, extreme. Not to mention a few obvious health risks to both mom and baby, or the fact that those women will not be around for many of their kids' milestone moments. I am not judging, but for me, seeing a geriatric physician and an obstetrician at the same time just does not sound appealing. I do not want to be seventy when my children are ten years old.

My personal opinions—and all those septuagenarian births—aside, there are real risks involved when you put off pregnancy until you are approaching (or have already reached) menopause. In fact, many fertility clinics have cutoff ages, after which they will not provide reproductive assistance. These ages vary; some more conservative clinics and doctors will not provide reproductive help to women using their own eggs after the age of forty-four, if only because these clinics and physicians do not want to promote treatment when the chances of success are low. Many doctors provide reproductive help using donor eggs up until the mid-fifties—an age the American Society of Reproductive Medicine recently approved as safe enough for attempting to carry a pregnancy; beyond that age, the health risks associated with pregnancy are deemed to be simply too great. Each clinic can pretty much decide for itself which age is appropriate, though you would not have to look very hard to find obstetricians who are speaking out against pregnancies occurring much after the age of natural menopause. Many find assisting women with late-in-life motherhood unethical, given the potential health risks involved (for both mother and child). In other words, it is pretty hard to "first do no harm" if you are exposing someone unnecessarily to higher rates of gestational diabetes, preeclampsia (a condition that causes high blood pressure in pregnant women), miscarriage, and more.

Let's take a moment to dig into some of those potential issues. While it is hard to assess one's risk of gestational diabetes—because diabetes is associated not just with age but also with race, BMI, genetics, diet, exercise, and a whole host of other factors—these general statistics below give an idea of its overall prevalence per 1,000 women:

AT AGE 20:   **22** in **1,000** women

AT AGE 25:   **36** in **1,000** women

AT AGE 30:   **51** in **1,000** women

AT AGE 35:   **67** in **1,000** women

AT AGE 40:   **84** in **1,000** women

And while gestational diabetes may sound like a pesky, temporary problem—typically it ends with the pregnancy, meaning it most often does not cause long-term effects—it can bring about significant complications. Gestational diabetes can result in stillbirth or, less serious, lead to overweight infants, which is not great for delivery (I mean you are already pushing an object the size of a cantaloupe through an opening the size of a lime, so jumbo-sizing that baby is not ideal, to say the least) or for the baby's future health. Gestational diabetes increases your chance of C-section, your baby's chance of getting injured during delivery or of experiencing preterm birth and respiratory distress syndrome, and raises the odds that your baby will suffer low blood sugar and type-two diabetes later in life.

Particularly concerning are the staggering miscarriage rates associated with older mothers:

AT AGE 20: **1** in **10** women miscarry

AT AGE 35: **1** in **5**

AT AGE 40: **1** in **3**

AT AGE 45: **1** in **2**

There are also concerns about the health of the baby to consider. The risk of chromosomal and genetic disorders sharply increases as a mother ages—specifically, as their eggs age:

AT AGE 20: **1** in **526** babies are born with chromosomal or genetic disorders

AT AGE 30: **1** in **385**

AT AGE 40: **1** in **66**

AT AGE 45: **1** in **21**

Finally, one specific chromosome disorder, Down syndrome, also becomes far more likely to occur as mothers age, which is one of the main reasons doctors recommend genetic testing for all mothers older than thirty-five. Here are the numbers on that:

AT AGE 25: **1** in **1,250** babies are born with Down syndrome

AT AGE 30: **1** in **1,000**

AT AGE 35: **1** in **400**

AT AGE 40: **1** in **100**

AT AGE 45: **1** in **30**

AT AGE 49: **1** in **10**

The culprit? As we age, so too do our eggs—resulting in malalignment and mistakes when the chromosomes pull apart after they have combined with the chromosomes from sperm during fertilization. Our aging bodies, in fact, barely factor into the equation; many doctors now believe that if a forty-two-year-old woman has no medical problems and is in good shape, she can theoretically experience a pregnancy just as easy as that of a younger woman. But that does *not* mean the forty-two-year-old's baby is not more likely to suffer from chromosomal abnormalities, thanks to her four-decade-year-old eggs. And therein, of course, lies the rub.

Now let's talk about what are referred to as peri- or postmenopausal pregnancies (women who have babies before, during, or after menopause, which may not even sound possible but is; it involves injecting yourself full of hormones to make the pregnancy stick, essentially "tricking" your body into preparing for pregnancy). These pregnancies carry more serious risks, even when a woman uses younger donor eggs.

But let's set aside these medical complications for the moment, and acknowledge the elephant in the room about late-in-life pregnancy. What happens once the baby comes? A mother in her sixties, no matter how fit and healthy, simply does not have the same ability to keep up with an energetic six- or seven-year-old as a younger mother would. My mother is in her late sixties, and I cannot imagine her trying to keep up with a small child. And let's consider what happens to those children as time passes. There is not a lot of data on this phenomenon yet because it is still very new, so I will use myself to illustrate my point. I am in my late thirties and, as I mentioned, my mom is in her late sixties. Let's assume she is not going to need serious health care until she is seventy-eight (actually, let's *pray* this is true). By then, I will be forty-eight, and hopefully in a position to better help her as she ages. But imagine if she had had me at, say, fifty-five. I would only be *twenty-three* when she hit seventy-eight. And I can tell you without a doubt that there was no way I would have been able to help her at that age. In fact, it would have put tremendous pressure on me—emotionally, logistically, and financially.

So all this being said, becoming a geriatric mama sounds about as appealing as eating your afterbirth, right? But wait. Do not make up your mind about how old is too old just yet. These questions are complicated; to every point, there is a counterpoint. And because my aim is not to convince you of anything one way or another—other than to beg you to be aware of your fertility earlier!—I am going to present both sides.

Let's first consider why women are waiting so long these days. I believe there are myriad cultural and societal reasons. One of my theories (and I admit I may have read this somewhere, but I fully subscribe) is that the delay is rooted at least partially in what is called economic infertility—in other words, the notion that babies are simply cost-prohibitive until your income hits six digits. I would argue that this is especially true for those women who live in major metropolitan cities. I ask you, as a Manhattanite of nearly fifteen years: who can afford to have children in a place like New York, San Francisco, or Los Angeles?

I was twenty-two when I moved to New York, and I earned about $27,000 at my first job. I survived, in large part, off the generosity of the men who took me out to dinner and the free breakfast provided every morning at my first ad agency job. (I used to take three bagels every day—one for breakfast, one for lunch, and one for dinner.) I nearly wept with joy when we had catered meetings. Without those sources of free food, I literally could not eat. That is, not if I wanted to pay my rent. This was pretty much the state of things for several years. Sure, my salary increased here and there, but I did not start making any real money until my late twenties—and even then, it was just enough to pay rent and actually begin purchasing my own groceries. In fact, it really was not until my early to mid thirties that I realized I could finally afford to have a well-rounded life *and* a child (though that was back when I was married; these days I would argue that even on my very healthy salary, a child would be a big financial burden, especially if I needed to pay for fertility treatments).

But economic infertility is not our only hurdle. Aside from the fact that most of us have to work for years before we make a comfortable income, we also want success beyond money. We want to find work that challenges and fulfills us—we want careers, not jobs. We want success beyond simple dollar signs. But success takes time, focus, and dedication. It requires sacrifice: instead of going out on dates and investing in relationships, we invest in making a living, burning the midnight oil, getting to the office before the boss and leaving after everyone else is long gone. I know that has been the case with me. I have never not "leaned in" because of the family I *might* have one day, as author and Facebook COO Sheryl Sandberg suggests many women do. I do not know any women who have. In fact, I lean in harder because I do not have kids, and often pick up the slack for those who do.

Across the board, every one of my friends spent their younger years just as driven. Alison did not even think about having kids until she was about thirty—she had been focused on her career. "I started thinking about it after grad school," she says. "I think it was a combination of finishing school [and] feeling like, *Gosh, I've done a lot of things I've wanted to do, from a professional sense. I have close to ten years' experience. I've done grad school, I've done all these things.* You hold that up against your friends, who are starting to get married and have kids, and that's a kind of reminder—one that hits you right in the face—that, oh yeah, you really want that too."

All that leaning in might get you a fantastic job—but it can also mean that husbands, partners, boyfriends, and babies fall by the way-side, only coming back into our lives once we have finally reached a certain level of stability. And that is how many of us find our-selves single and without babies in our thirties, forties, and beyond. In fact, Amelia even had to postpone her egg-freezing process by a few months because she was so busy at work. "I was pretty motivated by September 2015, and was planning to do it that November," she says. "But then work just exploded on me, and I was so mad and stressed. I was still trying to force November to be the right time, but I ended up pushing it back two months. I realized I was the only person I needed to answer to. And I was stressed out and worried, and I did not want to freeze stressed-out little eggs!"

I do not think this status quo is going to change any time soon. Women will keep working in challenging jobs, and life will continue to be expensive. So with that in mind, I urge you to ask yourself again: how old is too old?

Consider a woman I recently interviewed for this book, who asked not to be named. We can just call her My Girl-Crush, because she is. I have a huge amount of respect for her, not because I aspire to be a fifty-something-year-old first-time mother to a newborn, as she is (in fact, I have zero desire to be changing diapers at fifty), but because I admire the way she took control of her reproductive future early, at a time when egg freezing was only experimental. My Girl-Crush began freezing batches of eggs when she was thirty-eight, going through multiple cycles of egg freezing. That was more than twelve years ago, and back then, none of the reputable fertility clinics in

New York City would touch her ovaries, let alone her eggs, with a ten-foot pole. She was, they told her, simply too old. So she sought treatment elsewhere—she had to fly out of state to less conventional, potentially less reputable, clinics—to obtain her (roughly) sixty frozen eggs. She enlisted a very handsome, athletic male friend of hers to provide her with some quality sperm. And at the ripe "old" age of fifty, after several rounds of embryo transfers over the course of about eight years, My Girl-Crush finally gave birth to a beautiful, healthy, bouncing baby daughter.

Now, ladies, before you go getting any ideas about simply waiting until you are fifty to get started on your baby-making journey—all because My Girl-Crush has assuaged all your fears—it must be said that this woman is not normal. I do not mean that in a judgy, negative way. In fact, I say it out of admiration. She is your classic overachiever, right on down to her lady bits. She is highly successful, well-rounded, and, as I said, intimidatingly smart. She is also in amazing shape—she was a serious athlete as a younger woman and continues to stay very fit. She told me that while she was pregnant, the nurses and her doctor were constantly fawning all over her, half expecting her to drop dead or have serious complications. But nothing happened. All those complications I wrote about earlier never materialized for her. She had a smooth, healthy, perfectly normal pregnancy. But that certainly does not mean every fifty-year-old woman will.

When I visited My Girl-Crush at her fabulous apartment in one of the most coveted neighborhoods in Manhattan, she looked happy and, frankly, better at handling a newborn than many of my friends who had babies in their twenties. We chatted about her many cycles of egg freezing and her thoughts about becoming a first-time mother at her age. She said, wisely, that egg freezing is not the solution to all our problems but that more women should consider it, particularly if they are young. While she would have ideally had a baby when she was slightly younger, she points out that we are aging and maturing at a slower pace these days, staying healthier later into our golden years, and living much longer than ever before. So is having a baby at fifty really that crazy? To her, fifty is practically the new thirty.

It was surprising that My Girl-Crush brought up finances as a chief reason she waited so long to conceive. I guess, given the massive apartment we were sitting in when we had this chat, I had assumed finances had not been a concern of hers for quite some time. She told me that one of the benefits of having a baby at her age is that she is better off now than she has ever been, and continues to work in a lucrative field. Not only has she amassed a comfortable amount of money, she continues to have earning potential. Given her peak physical condition, she could conceivably be healthy for another thirty years! So she is financially secure and will continue to be, and she is healthy and happy, which is the ideal frame of mind for handling a demanding newborn. Her baby is lucky to have her as her mama, no matter how big the age gap between them.

As amazing as My Girl-Crush's story is, I have met very few women who aspire to emulate it. That is, few of us wish to become first-time moms at fifty. Yet, interestingly, I have noticed that among women without babies who want them eventually, the "acceptable" age to have a first child seems to increase as they age. In other words, my theory is that the older you get, the more open you are to having a baby later. (For some of my friends, that means postmenopausal pregnancy.) In my survey of about 150 women, I found that the older the woman surveyed, the older she said she could imagine being a first-time mother.

Also, it seems worth mentioning that, as Kate points out, fertility treatments can take a long time to be successful. "If you start thinking about this when you're thirty-five," she says, "there's a chance you'll not have your first child until you're nearly in your forties." That is something else to consider when mapping out the rest of your life.

As I write this, my thirty-eight-year-old self is very single. So at this not-so-prime baby-making age, what's my point of view on the question of how old is too old? I do not know for sure. What I do know is that I would like to make a decision soon, one way or the other. Because what is more important to me at this stage is not necessarily having a baby but knowing what I want, and knowing I will be happy with whatever decision I make, because it will be *my* decision rather than a sad eventuality.

Now, a disclaimer: your answer to the question of how old is too old is entirely an individual decision, which cannot be made lightly and should not be judged. All of this is to say, do not take my answer as gospel; I am just speaking about what I feel personally. And for me, the only way to preserve my own sanity is to make a decision and then move forward. I refuse to be one of these women who wish for a baby well into their forties and do nothing about it except hope to meet Mr. Right. Maybe I will meet him, or maybe I won't. I cannot let his arrival—or failure to arrive—be the deciding factor.

I know a lot of single women in their late forties who feel like they have simply run out of options, baby-wise. They have regrets. They pine over what they could have done differently, back when they had the chance. Then again, I also have friends in their late forties who could take babies or leave them, and are enjoying life with zero regrets. For example, Heather, who froze her eggs when she was thirty-eight, has decided she will either use them or lose them at forty-five. And while she admits that the latter outcome is a sad thought, she feels like she needs to set a limit for herself to avoid thinking *What if?* for the rest of her life. I admire that.

Lauren also has a great outlook on how to figure out if it is really the right time: go with your gut. "I'm thirty-eight, going to be thirty-nine soon," she says. "And I definitely feel my desires changing. I've been waiting for that to happen, and now it is. I think honestly it's a difference that came with age—not just the number but my physicality. Also, this might sound stupid, but I got a puppy about six months ago and it has been a great experience raising something, even if it is just a dog. I am longing for something more in life, and I think kids would be really great. I think emotionally I'm more ready, financially I'm more ready. I feel that it's time."

However, for those women who could not imagine a life in which they did not become a mother but now find themselves in their mid to late forties without children, being out of options is the worst and most heart-wrenching place to be. I hope never to experience that—that anger, resentment, and regret, that tiny bit of bitter man-hating. Though many of these women are killing it in other areas of their lives—running companies and running around town with friends, pursuing passion projects and traveling the world—and are not likely to sit around crying over babies they never had, they definitely experience a feeling of loss. We have figured out a lot in the world of fertility, but one thing we have not figured out yet is how to turn back time.

The question of how old is too old may not be something you can answer right away (I myself am still grappling with it, and I literally am writing the book on the subject), but at least you will be thinking about it. And when baby happens, or does not happen, it will be the result of a conscious decision you have made, not one you failed to make. When will you pull the trigger, and how might you view the decision to freeze your eggs? Which brings us to the next essential question to ask yourself.

2. Do I see freezing my eggs as an insurance policy— or a gamble?

I have often thought about whether or not the act of freezing my eggs was a kind of grown-up security blanket—an insurance policy to hedge against my future reproductive decline—or whether it was simply a big, fat gamble. Maybe it falls somewhere in the middle of these two extremes. Whatever the truth, and even if I never use my eggs, I will never for a minute regret my decision to freeze them. I believe that whether you see egg freezing as an insurance policy or a gamble is a question of optimism versus pessimism—a question, in other words, of seeing the uterus half full or half empty.

As we have discussed, the data on egg freezing success rates is a little all over the place. (Success, obviously, is defined as a live birth.) Egg freezing is still a relatively new procedure, so there are very few broad-stroke stats to help make your decision-making process cut-and-dried. It is hard to say just how many frozen eggs have led to live births, because clinics do not consistently report this data. Even if they did, the numbers are difficult to truly quantify: while more and more women are freezing their eggs, there is, obviously, a lag between the time they are frozen and the time they are used (if they are used at all). Many eggs have been frozen that have not yet been thawed for use, which skews the stats to a significant degree.

But what we do know is that doctors say the chance of a live birth resulting from one frozen egg is about 3 to 10 percent per egg, depending on our age, of course. (Not to fret, though: you typically get a lot more than one egg during an egg-freeze cycle. To put that stat in perspective, the chance for a live birth from IVF is about 6 percent per egg.) And there have been studies on success rates that suggest about 25 to 40 percent of women who freeze their eggs wind up having a baby. Not amazing, I know. If, at my job, I successfully carried out my objectives only 25 to 40 percent of the time, I likely would not have said job anymore.

There is also some evidence that suggests frozen eggs may not be as likely to result in pregnancy as fresh eggs. Doctors are not yet sure why, but it could be because freezing (and the subsequent thawing process) may actually diminish the quality of the eggs. There are statistics that seem to bear that out: In 2013, live birthrates were 56.1 percent for embryos made from fresh donor eggs and 47.1 percent for those made with frozen eggs. This suggests successful live births when using frozen eggs as opposed to fresh may be lower. (Though, keep in mind that donors tend to be young, which may have affected the outcome of those statistics.) Meanwhile, it is worth noting that doctors at NYU Langone Medical Center cite very different statistics—only about a 4 percent drop-off. It is important to appreciate that egg freezing and egg thawing performed on a large scale is a relatively new phenomenon and many clinics are not yet up to speed on technology. It behooves you to do some homework on the clinic you're considering, relative to how many treatment cycles they perform and how many babies they have created from thawed eggs. As you can see, there just is not yet a consensus in the medical community around this topic, in part because of the differences in the labs that freeze eggs. Ladies, we will just have to make the best, most informed decision possible.

Numbers are somewhat hard to go on anyway. What can you make of such statistics when every study yields a different result, and there are so many variables, such as the woman's general health, the sperm being used to fertilize the egg, and other factors? After reading all this, you might be leaning heavily toward the "this is a gamble" side of the spectrum—and who could blame you?

But let's try seeing that uterus as half full for a moment, and explore the other side of these seemingly dismal statistics. While the hard numbers may seem like nothing to write home about, Dr. Druckenmiller and Dr. Noyes recently told me that they and the other doctors at their institution absolutely believe that egg freezing *does* work, and can in fact yield healthy babies. They agree that the success rates may be so low because oocyte cryopreservation is still a relatively new procedure (at least as it relates to the masses, in its nonexperimental form). They reiterated that while a lot of women have frozen their eggs, they tend to leave them stored for several years at a time, if not indefinitely. Which means the data is far more delayed than most medical data.

Even more heartening, there have been some promising studies in recent years, each of which indicates a far higher success rate than the ones I mentioned previously. These studies suggest that if you are using eggs that were frozen at age thirty-four or younger, the chances of a live birth with those eggs was closer to 50 percent.

Additionally, according to the Los Angeles Fertility Center, 5,000 babies have been born from frozen eggs, and as far as doctors can tell, babies born of frozen eggs are just as healthy (accounting for the age of the eggs used) as they would be had they been born from fresh eggs. The largest study of these babies (reported by Dr. Noyes), which tracked about 900 of the 5,000 born from frozen eggs, showed there was no increased rate of birth defects when compared to the general population.

While 5,000 babies worldwide does not seem like a big, convincing statistic, keep in mind that this is a new procedure, and most women who have frozen their eggs have not yet returned to thaw them. The important thing to remember is that egg freezing is simply a new technology, and while we know it *can* work, we do not fully know yet to what extent. The truth is, we probably will not know that for years, when women start to return to the clinics and thaw their eggs to attempt to get pregnant.

So back to the question at hand: is egg freezing a risky gamble or a wise insurance policy? Let's define our terms. "Insurance" involves guaranteed protection against a potential eventuality. And, strictly speaking, egg freezing cannot be that—because, I am sorry to say, there are no guarantees to be found here. The process may work, and it may not. So set aside your belief that freezing your eggs will be a silver bullet, a failsafe, a reassuring certainty. This is your classic *que sera, sera* situation: whatever will be, will be. That's life, as they say.

To "gamble," on the other hand, is to risk losing something of value in order to potentially gain something of greater value. In the case of egg freezing, the potential loss is about twenty grand. But the gain is a human life—the human life you have so badly wanted to create, perhaps for years. Perhaps for your entire life. The gain is also becoming a mom.

Even if egg freezing is a gamble—and it does seem to be, based on these definitions—for me it was well worth the risk. The potential gain is so much greater than the potential loss. And without that gamble, I may not get the chance to have a baby at all. Even with egg freezing's not-so-impressive supposed 25 to 40 percent success rate—a number that varies wildly based on such factors as age and number of eggs retrieved—I think we would all agree that this procedure can offer some hope.

The way my friends feel about egg freezing varies. Alison, for example, says, "I thought, *I will kick myself later on in life if I don't do this*. I know it isn't a guarantee, I know there are a lot of variables. But I want to know that I will be able to look back and say I did everything I could to give myself a choice. There are so many things that we can't control, but this is something I *can* control. I thought, *Well, here's one choice you actually can make*. The feeling of that is unbelievable."

She also feels it has positively influenced her dating life. "I feel like I really can wait for the right person," Alison says. "If I didn't have the eggs, I could see myself thinking about settling, meeting someone and thinking, *Sure, this will work*. But I think now I've granted myself the possibility of waiting until something is really right."

3. Am I making this choice out of fear?

In talking about the subjects of egg freezing and fertility with so many women, I have observed a curious coincidence. (Or maybe it is not a coincidence at all—you be the judge.) Many of us start thinking about freezing our eggs after a bad breakup. If you think about it, the logic makes perfect sense: we thought this person might be the father of our theoretical children, and now that he's gone, we realize just how difficult it could be to find the right guy for that role. Sometimes the greatest pain of a breakup is that we thought we were all set—that the crucial decisions that would bring us to our happily-ever-after had already been made, and now we could relax. We had the guy, we had the strong foundation, we had put in the necessary time, and now talking about kids was appropriate. Once that "all-set" situation falls apart through a breakup or divorce, the realization that we have to start all over can be terrifying. The clock is suddenly set back to zero hundred hours, but we do not have as much time as we did when said relationship first started. Ergo, we start counting down the time we have left to procreate, and many of us make our way to the egg-freezing clinic. Who can blame us?

A few of my friends have lived this phenomenon. Alison, for example, got serious about egg freezing after a tough breakup—actually, after two breakups. "I had my tests done when I was thirty-one," she says. "I got my results, and they were not fabulous. That threw me into *what now?* mode. I was considering freezing my eggs, but I thought, *I'll sit on it for a bit.* Then I met a guy, and he became my boyfriend. I decided to hold off on the procedure. He and I dated for a year and a half, but it didn't work out. I was thirty-two by then. Six months after we ended things, I decided to have the tests redone. *Let's see what's happened in a year.* Sure enough, the numbers had dropped even more." That was when she went forward with the procedure.

When I asked Amelia when she started to think more concretely about her fertility, she had this to say: "I think it was probably around when I was thirty-one. That was when I started to have a new vision of myself as an adult. I was unhappy with the life I had. I was unfulfilled in my relationship and in my job, and I was having family issues with my parents and sisters. I fell into this hole, and I didn't know how to dig my way out. I really felt like I needed to make some changes in my life. It took therapy and working toward finding something new to finally feel like I was on the right track. There are only so many things you can control in your life, and I knew my job and my relationship were among them. The relationship I was in ended, and I looked at my job at the time, and I looked at the fact that I was single at thirty-one and wasn't going to get married any time soon. Which meant I wasn't going to have kids any time soon. I thought,

How old will I be when I do meet someone? That was when I started thinking about freezing my eggs."

Amelia also told me a heart-wrenching story about a friend of hers. "A few years ago, she went through the same thing I did," she says. "She found herself in a breakup with the man she thought she would be married to and building a family with. She said, 'I'm going to do it right now,' meaning freeze her eggs, and she went in to see the doctor, and they were like, 'There's really nothing left.' She was thirty-four, and she had no eggs. I would have been heartbroken. That's a tough pill to swallow."

Listen, there is absolutely nothing wrong with thinking about freezing your eggs after a breakup or divorce. I mean, obviously I would feel that way—it is, after all, exactly what I did. But there *is* something to be said for not making decisions based in panic. I waited a while after my divorce before I finally went through with the procedure. The problem with panic is that it makes us rash. It breeds recklessness, impulsiveness, poor judgment. It clouds the issue we are weighing. So what we often wind up doing is making the choice that most quickly and effectively quells our panic, which is not necessarily the same thing as the *right* choice.

Decide whatever you want, of course. You have every right to make this decision whenever and however and under whatever circumstances you like. Maybe your breakup—or another source of baby-making anxiety—is just the push you need to start thinking more concretely about your fertility. If so, more power to you. I just think it is important to caution against making decisions *solely* out of fear. That rarely ends well for anyone.

In fact, what I would love to see more of is this decision being made as a normal part of what you do in your twenties. It should be a purely objective and proactive decision—a decision made because you were well informed about your reproductive health and still had the option to do something about it—and not the reaction to a circumstance that has you suddenly worried about your fertility.

4. Am I willing to do the whole single mom thing?

Even as recently as a few years ago, I would never have considered having a baby outside of marriage, let alone having one solo. For me, like for so many women, the equation was simple and unwavering: Family = Me (adored wife) + Man (handsome, successful husband) + Bouncy Baby (or Babies). But things have changed since then. I got older, basically, and realized a few things about myself and also about relationships. Now that I do not think I want to be a wife again, and given that I think I want to be a mom, it leads to the natural conclusion that I may have to be okay with being a *single* mom.

Some of my friends are coming to that very same conclusion. Others say they will never be single moms. While Heather certainly has the means to have a child on her own if she wanted to, when I spoke to her about being a single mom, she said she had zero interest. "I was raised by a single mom," she says. "My dad wasn't a huge part of my life. While my mom did an amazing job, it's not something I really aspire to do." Heather is keeping her frozen eggs safely stored until she meets someone. And if she never meets anyone, she will donate her eggs to science or sell them, assuming that becomes legal and there is a market for so-called "old eggs" (sorry, Heather, you were no spring chicken when you froze them!).

On the other hand, Heidi says she would have no problem parenting alone if she suddenly found that animal instinct to mother, which has not really happened for her. "Am I opposed to saying someday I'll do this on my own?" she asks. "Totally unopposed to that. I think that's fine. I think family comes in all sorts of forms. I have enough of a network around me, I have enough of an extended family that that kid would have a family. So I think that's a totally viable option."

Similarly, Victoria always knew she would be fine with doing the mom thing alone—which is exactly what she now does. "My plan was basically that if I had not met anyone by the time I was forty,

I would do it on my own. That was a huge decision, which I made when I was about thirty-five. But deciding on that plan so early on gave me time to live with it, to talk to my family about it, to get comfortable with it."

On the opposite end of the spectrum, Alison struggles mightily with the possibility of becoming a single mom. In fact, when I asked her if she would ever go it alone, she began to cry. "I can't really answer that question," she said through her tears. "I think I'm pretty dead set and hopeful and positive that it'll work out so I can use these eggs with a partner. But I think if it gets to a certain point and that hasn't happened, and the desire to have children is becoming more and more relevant to me, I will be glad to know I have these. I haven't spent a ton of time thinking about it, because—I won't lie—that's not what I hope will happen. I really hope it isn't. But I think I will know I'm ready when I know. For right now, I'm hopeful that that's not what's in my future."

The reality of single parenthood also gives Amelia pause. "If at forty I'm still single," she says, "I would consider starting the implantation process then. But that would mean I would have to save up for that, and also save up to be a single mom. I don't know how I would do that. I don't know how anyone does that. It's tough."

Those are sobering words—and I think about many of the same things. I am frightened by the difficulty of raising a child on a single income, and by the hell of knowing that when that baby cries during the night, only you are there to comfort her.

If you are in your twenties or early thirties, you may not believe you may someday have to ask yourself the single-mom question. Then again, maybe you will not ever have to ask it at all. Maybe you are involved with someone who will turn out to be the father of your children, or maybe you are happily single but will eventually meet someone who will be that father. But—and I do not mean to scare you, I promise—there is a chance you will not, especially if you live in New York City, where so many men have that Peter Pan syndrome (thanks to living on an island of beautiful, accomplished women who are all ripe for the picking).

If I sound jaded, I promise you I am not—I am simply making the best of my reality. A very wise woman put this all in perspective for me not too long ago. I was talking to her about this book and about my journey with fertility in general, and she said, "Why don't you just have a baby on your own? Men are pretty useless with babies anyway, which means you end up taking care of *two* babies!" She was serious. I was stunned. I do not consider myself naive, but when we had this conversation—and seriously, it was not that long ago—I still believed there was a good chance I would find a partner to have a family with. It was hard to hear such a frank acknowledgment that I might not.

She went on. "You're pretty, smart, accomplished, blah, blah. You're all the things people point out when they wonder why you're still single," she said, "but none of that matters." She pointed out that at my age, most of the men in my peer group are either already married or are not married because they do not want to be. (Again, there is that Peter Pan syndrome I mentioned.) Older men, whom I have tended to go for in the past, are typically divorced—often with children, meaning they are most likely not interested in doing the baby thing all over again. This wise woman I was speaking to happens to be friends with the man I was involved with at the time, and she very bluntly told me not to hold my breath for him to come around. (In the end, she turned out to be right.) I left our conversation feeling enlightened and more than a little empowered. Why *couldn't* I just do this baby thing on my own?

I have only ever been in one relationship where having a child was on the table, and that was with my ex-husband. I have been out of that relationship for about three years now. I have had relationships here and there since then. I even fell in love once—with the man I mentioned previously. Obviously that did not work out. Even as I see myself running out of time, I continue to pick the wrong guys. And I have to ask myself: *Am I really going to change? Or should I just admit that I like a certain type of man—the type who does not really want to settle down or have kids—and decide that is fine, because I am independent and I can, if I want to, have a baby on my own?*

Soon after my separation from my ex-husband, I fell for that man I just mentioned. He thoroughly swept me off my feet. He was the funniest, smartest, most charming and insightful person I had ever met—and still is. He knew me better than I knew myself within minutes of meeting me! After just a few weeks together, I felt like he knew me, and "got me," better than anyone else in my life. We spent almost a year together. A crucial year. It would probably have been better spent finding a relationship with someone who wanted the same things or, instead, coming to terms with the possibility of being a single mom.

It was the sad but necessary ending of this relationship that taught me to stop relying on a man for certain things. While I had never relied on men for much, I had, up until that point, assumed I would need one to become a mother. But at the time of this breakup, I started to ask myself whether or not I could separate my desire to be a mother from my desire to be loved by a man—especially if that man did not want any kids (or any *more* kids). The man I had been seeing was nearly fifty. His child was well on her way to adulthood. It was fair enough that he did not want to revisit the diaper-changing, baby-chasing, sleepless-nights phase of his life. Two facts presented themselves: One, I loved him. Two, I had the emotional, psychological, and financial capacity to have a baby on my own. So why couldn't he fulfill my romantic desires while I had a baby solo? Well, with this particular man, that wasn't possible, because his not wanting a child was not our only problem; he simply did not want a relationship, period.

But couldn't that setup—me as a single mom, romantically involved with a man—work with some other, future man? I think it could. Heidi and I spoke about this recently. "I would love for there to be more counternarratives in our culture about women and having children," she says. "I'm thirty-seven, I'm single, I don't have kids, I don't really want to have kids, I consider myself a decently strong personality, and *still* it's hard to overcome the cultural narrative of all those rom-coms we watch, and *Say Yes to the Dress*, and the perfect wedding, and all the Pinterest stuff—there's so much pressure on us to conform that I don't think we even realize it. I felt it when I stopped conforming to it, when I had to start listening to myself. Part of my ability to listen to myself was to freeze the eggs and divorce myself from the emotional narrative around having kids. I think that was a key part of understanding who I am as a human being, not just as a woman. If you want to fall in love when you're young and have three kids by the time you're twenty-six, cool, that's totally fine. But can we create alternative narratives? I think freezing your eggs is part of that."

I do think separating romance from baby could be a good thing— for me, and possibly for us all. It takes the pressure off, because God knows when you are dating in your late thirties or even forties, most men assume you are viewing them through the filter of baby-daddy potential. If I can afford to do the baby thing on my own, why make every date a daddy audition? Beyond the fact that seeing men this way kills the fun and romance of dating, the reality is, as I have seen with a few close friends who are new moms, there are a few men who can be pretty useless when it comes to helping with a baby. Once they contribute their swimmers, the rest is often like pulling teeth. (Sorry, men, I know this is a huge generalization, but I am seeing more and more women who are bringing home the bacon, frying it up in the pan, and then being forced to wash the pan afterward because you could not be bothered to. Not cool.)

So let's consider—just for argument's sake, no need to panic!— the pros and cons of being a single mom:

PROS:

- You pick your specimen without any emotional attachment. I have, as I mentioned, been browsing sperm bank sites, and I have to say, it is amazingly liberating when the only thing you need from a man is semen. I am just going on physical appearance, intelligence levels, and medical history. Honestly, I wish I could be this objective about men I get into relationships with.

- You only have the baby (or babies) to take care of. Some men can be quite needy, as you have probably realized by now—and do you *really* want yet another needy creature around when you already have one keeping you up all night and relying on your body for sustenance? Sadly, I have heard from many women whose husbands or boyfriends weren't half as helpful as they had hoped when it came to those early days of fatherhood. In some cases—the worst of the worst dads—their men actually created *more* work. That is a pain no woman with a newborn needs.

- You can raise your child however you like. No squabbling over religion, what school they go to, what sports they do and do not play, or what they are allowed and not allowed to eat. You get the gist. You are in control, and you answer to no one but yourself. Sounds pretty good to me.

- You are actively redefining what family looks like. You will be raising a child or children who will grow up seeing a version of life where divorce or singledom does not cripple or tear families apart, where a woman does not need a man to survive or to pursue her deepest desires, and where parents can be independent people, choosing to be in a relationship when it is working and done with that relationship when it is not. In other words, you will be raising a child who learns never to settle. And you will be helping to write another, newer, more modern narrative of what is acceptable and "normal" when it comes to how women choose to live their lives. That is pretty cool.

CONS:

- There's the whole "crushing financial and logistical burden of raising a child on your own" thing. Just, you know, *that*.

- While some men might suck at the baby thing, they do come in pretty handy. Even I have to admit that having a strong father figure is important. While I did not grow up in a traditional family—my parents went through a very ugly divorce when I was seven—both my biological father and my stepdad played pivotal roles in my life. My real dad and I were not particularly close while I was growing up, but in adulthood, I learned to respect his work ethic, his focus, his ability to run his business, and his commitment to his new family. I learned from him that objective decision making is the key not just to success but also to life. My stepdad, who was in many ways a very different person than my dad, was the ultimate family man. He stuck by my mom's side through thick and thin, and took in her two children even though he already had two of his own (plus, they had another child together!). So I was lucky to have two father figures. Neither was a traditional dad, but they each taught me different things. Jump back for a moment to the "Pros" column, the key word here is "figure"—in other words, this person in your child's life does not literally have to be your child's dad.

- You can raise your child however you like. Yes, I know this was also one of the pros—and the freedom to direct your parenting plan does have some major upsides. But think about this for a second. With no twenty-four-hour sounding board, no partner in the process, you have nobody to help you make some of the really important decisions. Of course, you can read parenting books and ask your pediatrician and your mom and your friends—but they will not always be there when the kid is screaming his head off at four in the morning and you are not sure how to calm him down, and they cannot tell you with any real authority whether you should take your kid to church or public school or flute lessons. In the end, that is always going to be your call and your call alone. If you have a partner, you share the weight of that burden.

- You will not have someone to play good cop / bad cop with. You will be all cops. Every cop, every time. You will be the nurturer *and* the disciplinarian. The math tutor and the creator of Halloween costumes (even if you are awful at math and never learned how to sew). And as I have learned in other aspects of my life, when you try to take on too many things, you might wind up not doing any of them well.

Confession: I honestly had a harder time coming up with the cons of being a single mom than the pros. And while the cons are definitely biggies, none of them are what keep me personally from taking the plunge. I have not gone for single momhood yet because—okay, I admit, here is one more con—getting pregnant without a man to knock you up is a logistical and financial nightmare.

As I mentioned, a few months ago, after a three-year hiatus, I began talking to my fertility doctor again—this time about starting fertility treatments on my own. My insurance claimed to cover them, so I thought at least the finances of it would be less of a burden. My doctor advised me to start with IUI, and if that did not work after five cycles, she would move me up to IVF. It sounds simple, but at the time, my day job plus writing this book made it *very* difficult for me to get away for the myriad appointments, for the blood work, for running around to pick up my various drugs. I simply did not have time to get pregnant that way. Oh, and just so you know, when you are a single woman using donor sperm, some clinics make you undergo a psychological evaluation to make sure you understand the implications of your decision and the amount of responsibility that comes with the procedure—a paternalistic precaution, if you ask me. Why do they need to make sure *I am sane* while miserable couples halfway to divorce can procreate at will? (Not to mention that the psychological evaluation was just another appointment I did not have time for.)

I know what you are thinking: if I do not have time to get pregnant, how do I expect to have time to be a mom? But hear me out. If I could get pregnant the old-fashioned way, I would make an amazing mom. Busy, preoccupied women get pregnant all the time, and when the baby comes, they manage to juggle it or slow down—they figure it out. I would too. But I have the added burden of doing this artificially, which requires a great deal of time and, as I soon found out, money.

Because guess what! Even if your insurance program covers fertility treatments, they can make it very difficult for you to take advantage of these benefits if you are single.

We talked about this briefly already, but here I will break it down further. I had foolishly signed up for the most expensive insurance plan my company offers, because it claimed to cover fertility treatments. And it does—provided you are married and have been trying to get pregnant with your husband for a specified period of time. (Even more on my thoughts about the healthcare industry and fertility later, because this topic warrants its own chapter, believe me.)

So here is where things stand: I have no time for the treatments at the moment. I cannot afford to pay the thousands of dollars it costs per treatment (including drugs, the procedure, all of the blood work and monitoring, and also the cost of the baby batter). I mean, maybe I could afford it *once*, but knowing it will most likely take anywhere from three to five embryo transfers to get pregnant, that is an enormous financial commitment. (Say I end up paying on the high side of that range, and I get lucky and the process takes me just three cycles, I will likely have shelled out about $45,000 for a child before he or she is even born—more on the cost breakdown later—and I still have the rest of its life to go.) I am just not able to take that on right now.

Which brings me to one option we have not mentioned yet—perhaps the simplest one of all, in theory. I can just go find a man willing to get me pregnant, no strings attached, right? Actually, that is more difficult than you might expect. A few male friends of mine—some straight, some gay—have offered up their sperm, which is a very generous offer indeed. But if I took them up on it, I would still have to go through IUI, unless we just went for it and had sex—and given that we would almost certainly have to do it more than once, that is kind of a commitment. (And kind of an awkward commitment, at that.) Not to mention the added complication of being forever tied to a man who is not my partner, and who might potentially want to be in the baby's life. That could definitely complicate things.

Or I could just hold out for a partner who wants the same things in life. But that is like quitting your job because you might someday win the lottery. Yes, it *could* happen, but do you really intend to go broke waiting? I do not.

There is yet another option—one I have been toying with a lot lately—which is forgoing motherhood if things do not play out as planned. When I started writing this book, I was, to be frank, obsessed with figuring out how I would become a mother one day. I still *think* I want that, but I am also starting to step into my stride. Not to mention that I have seen some of my girlfriends struggle with babies either as single women or with needy partners. While I sometimes look at their babies with envy, I also know my friends often wish they had my life instead of the headaches children bring.

So after all these considerations—after all the thinking and weighing and comparing and list making—let me sum up. Would I do the mom thing alone? I still have no clue. But I do think it is worth asking yourself the question. In fact, I think it is essential.

5. Is having children really what I want?

This may be the trickiest question of them all. It can feel nearly impossible to untangle your own feelings from what your culture, your parents, or your friends tell you to feel about potential parenthood. You might not think so—you are tough, smart, used to knowing (and getting) what you want. Of course, you know whether or not you want to have kids. But consider this: the way in which our culture telegraphs to us that our womanhood is only truly complete when we have become mothers is so subtle, so insidious, that even the toughest and most clear-eyed among us can fall under its sway.

Furthermore, we women are faced with time pressures that can cloud that decision even more. In your mid thirties or so, if you do not already have kids, you inevitably start getting questions: "So when do you think you'll settle down and start a family?" And the question of "when" presupposes the "if"—it assumes, in other words, that having a child is, *of course*, the next phase of your life, the only way to complete your journey. The question implies that having children is the only way to pass time between being young and being old. And so you start to panic, and you fill in the blanks with what society expects: that, as a woman, you will become a mother. And you'd better get a move on!

When I asked my friends if they were *sure* they wanted to have kids—and how they knew for sure—I received a fascinating array of answers. "Yes, a hundred percent," said Alison. "I have always, always been passionate about and driven to have children. I think it has always been top of mind for me. With that said, I am also driven from a professional standpoint as well. But I've never treated it as an either/or situation—like, 'If I choose to have kids, I need to stop that,' or 'If I continue to try and grow my professional identity, I will have to put kids on the back burner.' I want both, and I think I can *have* both. I've always said that I will continue to build my career, but if I meet the right person, having a baby will edge its way up my list of priorities."

Amelia was more ambivalent. I asked her, too, if she had always wanted to have children. "I think so," she said. "I think it was something I always assumed would happen. I never really thought about it either way, to be honest. I think it was more that I just envisioned it as part of my life, once I was an adult."

Lauren had a very different answer. "No, definitely not," she said. "I mean, I also wasn't sure that I *didn't* want to have them—I just wasn't a hundred percent sure either way. I never had that strong maternal drive that I think a lot of my friends had, and certainly did not have it at a young age. I was actually always a little worried that I just did not have that drive . . . did that mean I didn't want to have kids? I felt the same about a wedding, or a marriage: I just never really imagined the wedding dress followed by a house in the suburbs and the white picket fence. That was just never really me. I would rather be off traveling the world and having amazing life experiences."

Meanwhile, Victoria said simply, "Yes. Always." Kate was similarly sure: "Yes," she said, "but I didn't experience it as a burning when I was younger—I didn't feel it as a burning desire. I always assumed I would have children, back in my twenties. But there were a lot of things I had burning desires for that came higher on the list." Ana also never questioned whether she would be a mother. "That desire actually has always been a given," she says. "I always kind of assumed that I would. I think when I imagined a future it was easier to imagine children than it was a partner, in fact."

Heidi summed up perfectly the kind of forced decision making that plagues so many of us. (Heidi, as you know, decided she might not be so keen on having children after all, but only once she had frozen her eggs.) "I had always envisioned myself as someone who would be a mom," she says. "But I don't think that was an active choice; it was more of a cultural choice—'Of course, this is going to happen someday,' that kind of thing." Falling prey to ambient pressure floating on the air is deceptively easy. And it happens to the best of us.

How, then, can you gauge whether you truly want children—or if you only think you do? Sometimes it will be easy. Sometimes your gut feeling will make itself known, whispering and then speaking and then shouting until you finally get the message. That was certainly how it was for Kate. "My sister got married much earlier than

I did, settled down younger, and had kids in her late twenties," she says. "We grew up very close, so without thinking much about it I'd always had this assumption that my kids and hers would grow up together. And the older her children got, and the more I enjoyed them, I began to imagine that same situation for myself. It wasn't my top ambition, but then my sister having kids made it a lot more of a positive vision rather than an assumption. I became more and more conscious of the fact that they were growing up and I didn't have kids yet. My sister's kids became these little human calendars, reminding me of the passage of time."

For other women, the answer to this question is harder to discern. If that describes you, I advise you to look at it from every (hypothetical, imaginary, made-up) angle. Imagine how you would feel if you found out you had no choice in the matter whatsoever, that a doctor looked you in the eye and said it would never happen. Imagine how you would feel if someone gave you all the money you would need to raise a happy, healthy kid, or all the time or space. If you can imagine having zero impediments to having a child—if the circumstances were 100 percent perfect—and you still are not sure it is right for you, that tells you something. If you can imagine ardently wanting a child despite having none of those things in place, that tells you something too. Figuring this out is not easy. But it is much easier if you are aware early, and if you give yourself options by, for example, freezing your eggs. What is also helpful is telling yourself over and over, and spreading the word, that whether or not you want to be a mom is your choice and no one else's.

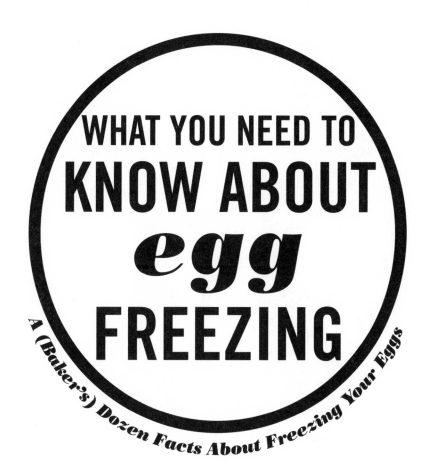

WHAT YOU NEED TO KNOW ABOUT *egg* FREEZING

A (Baker's) Dozen Facts About Freezing Your Eggs

N ow that you have the lay of the land—the stone-cold facts about your fertility timeline and the skinny on how your hardware works—you may be wondering more seriously if egg freezing might be the way to go. That is great, of course. I am all for it! But before you get too excited, there are still a few things you should know. In fact, in this chapter we will cover a (baker's) dozen facts about freezing your eggs that any potential mother hen should be aware of.

Egg freezing is something, I would wager, that you have probably been hearing more about lately. Why, suddenly, does it seem like everyone is running out to freeze her eggs? What has suddenly pushed this technology into the limelight and, by extension, into the minds of lady urbanites all over the world? Two big parts of that are availability and acceptance. As women choose to start families later and later, the demand for workable fertility solutions has increased. Increased demand engenders a greater supply. And so we find ourselves here, living in a world where pregnancies made possible by scientific intervention are, at least in most major cities, Starbucks-level ubiquitous. As the cultural acceptance of such technology has become more widespread, that technology has become more available.

The science of egg freezing has only recently become sophisticated and developed enough for the American Society for Reproductive Medicine to stop referring to it as "experimental" and give the go-ahead for doctors and clinics to provide the service as an "elective" treatment for patients healthy (and financially equipped) enough to undergo the procedure. This technology is now available to anyone who can pay for it.

These landmark advancements in oocyte cryopreservation, coupled with an increased cultural and societal demand for fertility treatments and other fertility-preserving measures, have led to a lot of chatter about, and demand for, egg freezing in recent years. For most of us, including myself, this technology is an invaluable means to preserve our fertility and therefore extend our future options. Having this technology at our disposal is one of the purest forms of my notion of Birth Control 2.0, in which "control" does not just mean prevention but also the ability to fully command our future reproductive potential. What a time to be alive!

And with that, let's dive right into everything you need to know in order to make the most informed decision possible about your potential egg-freezing journey.

1. A brief history of egg freezing

Because this practice has been such a hot topic of late, you might be surprised to find out that sperm and embryos have long—and successfully—been frozen and later thawed. In fact, the first child conceived with frozen sperm was born in 1953. However, doctors and scientists had been trying to freeze sperm long before the 1950s. Some of these attempts were for agricultural purposes, and those early attempts did, in fact, yield healthy births (sure, they were animal babies—but babies nonetheless). Interest in freezing sperm was not limited to livestock: early attempts to freeze human sperm arose even before we possessed a full awareness of the effects that aging has on male fertility. In 1866, a man by the name of Montegazza was the first to consider the application of freezing human sperm, suggesting that "a man dying on a battlefield may beget a legal heir with his semen frozen and stored at home." It took a while to perfect the process, to say the least. While that first birth resulting from frozen sperm occurred in 1953, the first child born from a frozen embryo was not delivered until 1984, and the first child born from an egg frozen on its own (as opposed to being one half of a frozen embryo) was in 1986. That is a difference of more than thirty years.

Why such a long lag? It is a matter, in the end, of degrees of difficulty. While sperm is easy to access and freeze, and embryos are relatively easy to freeze, eggs are neither easy to extract nor to freeze. The production of multiple eggs requires hormones, and retrieving these eggs requires surgery; the production and retrieval of sperm involves little more than privacy and a Dixie cup.

Doctors have been successfully freezing and thawing embryos for years, with the first birth reported in 1984 and more than 500,000 babies born to date. Eggs on their own, however, have for decades proved to be far more difficult to freeze. They are, after all, pesky, fragile little things, thanks to the large amount of fluid they contain. When frozen, that fluid can expand and form ice crystals, damaging the cell membrane and the structure of the egg. Thus, crystallization is considered the biggest danger for the survival and viability of a frozen egg.

There are two methods for completing the egg-freezing process: the slow-freeze method, which has been used for decades to freeze embryos, and vitrification, which is thought to result in higher success rates (though the jury is still out on these methods' efficacy relative to each other).

In both methods, excess fluid in the eggs is removed, while what is known as a cryoprotectant is injected into the cells to minimize damage during the freezing and thawing processes. The combinations of cryoprotectants have been fine-tuned over the years, with success greater today than even five years ago.

In the slow-freeze method, the temperature is lowered very—you guessed it—slowly, while in vitrification the egg is frozen in a flash and stored in almost unfathomably cold liquid nitrogen. Actually, if you want to get *really* precise, during the slow-freeze method the temperature is lowered at the rate of less than 1°C per minute before freezing to –196°C in liquid nitrogen. Vitrification, on the other hand, brings the eggs to –196°C at a staggering rate of around -25,000°C per minute. That is not a tortoise-and-hare situation—that is more like a tortoise versus a supersonic jet.

While the advancement of egg freezing was largely triggered by a growing cultural desire to delay first pregnancies, the specific development of vitrification came about thanks to a very different source of social pressure: the strictures of religion-based Italian law. I know, that sounds strange, right?—but I will explain. Italian legislation relating to fertility is deeply rooted in the beliefs of the Catholic Church, meaning that matters of reproductive health and fertility are heavily influenced by the question of when life begins. Between 2003 and 2009, the Italian government imposed very strict limitations on how embryos were to be treated, and how many a couple was allowed to own. Embryos were legally considered to be tiny human beings— life begins at fertilization, according to the Catholic faith—and were to be treated as such. So when a couple sought fertility treatment, and it came time to inseminate their eggs during an IVF cycle, only three were permitted to be fertilized, and, once this was done, all three of these embryos had to be transferred to the woman's uterus in order to get the chance to fulfill their potential for life. Embryos were not to be frozen—if they were humans, the logic went, how could they just be put on ice, never allowed to blossom into a human life?

Eggs, on the other hand, being only half the human equation and therefore possessing no potential for life in and of themselves, *were* allowed by the Italian government to be frozen, presumably to ensure that when women produced more than the three eggs allowed for fertilization, those eggs would not be discarded. (Again, it is no easy feat producing a batch of mature eggs, let alone getting those suckers out—so every little egg helps.) But because freezing eggs had hardly been a smashing success in those early days of the slow-freeze process, scientists and doctors were incentivized to figure out a more effective means of preserving these unfertilized oocytes. Which is how the process of vitrification came about. Since then, Italy has lifted the limits on egg and embryo freezing, and a lot of scientific advancements have been made at clinics all over the world. Italy remains one of the world leaders in fertility medicine, as a result of their race to improve egg freezing over the last two decades.

With those advancements came wider acceptance. In 2012, the American Society for Reproductive Medicine (ASRM) lifted the experimental label from egg freezing, making the procedure much more widely available to women in the United States.

I am obviously not the only person who has taken advantage of these advances. While the procedure has become widely available—in that anyone who can afford to can access the technology —the number of women in the United States who have frozen their eggs is still relatively small but is very quickly growing, especially in metropolitan areas like New York, Los Angeles, San Francisco, and Chicago. According to reports from the Society of Assisted Reproductive Technology, the number of women freezing their eggs skyrocketed from 475 in 2009 to nearly 5,000 in 2013, and I am sure by now, that number has increased even more sharply (exact and current numbers are hard to come by because not all clinics report such statistics to the Society for Assisted Reproductive Technology). And demand is growing. EggBanxx, a Prodigy-owned company famous for their egg-freeze parties, brokering discounts between patients and clinics, and for providing loans to women who can't shell out tens of thousands of dollars for the procedure, estimates that by 2018, 75,000 women will have frozen their eggs.

While egg freezing certainly hasn't achieved the mass breakthrough that the birth control pill has (not yet, anyway), it has already garnered a great deal of media attention—good and bad. Some praise it. Some call it ethically complicated. Others attempt to portray it as some sexy new trend all women in the know ought to partake in, like micro pleats or contouring. Hell, some have even tried to turn egg freezing into a theme for parties, which come complete with martinis on rooftop bars and lame, winking puns about "freezing the clock." (No, I am not joking. More on these crimes against cryopreservation—and good taste—in a moment.)

So what exactly does this miraculous procedure entail? Let me explain it in a nutshell. (Actually, make that an eggshell.) Given the long technological and scientific history I just described, egg freezing probably sounds pretty complicated. And while there is definitely some serious science behind the methodology, in terms of what the procedure means for *you*, it is all really quite simple.

As I mentioned in the earlier overview of your lady bits, your body normally releases one egg per month. However, when you go through an egg-freezing cycle, the goal is to get your body to produce multiple eggs at the same time. This is accomplished through the use of daily hormone injections (the exact number and type depends on your body's response to the drugs you are prescribed). Your body generates a batch of eggs that mature until the time when you would normally ovulate. At this point, rather than your ovaries being left to release these eggs, the group generated is extracted with a needle in a procedure called an egg retrieval. The extracted eggs are then frozen in time via the high-tech freezing process of vitrification that I described.

Then, when you are ready to use the eggs you have frozen— perhaps a year later, perhaps a decade later (most data suggests that eggs can be frozen indefinitely without incurring any damage)—you go through the in vitro fertilization and embryo transfer process. Which means your eggs are thawed, then injected with sperm (be it your partner's or a donor's) in hopes that they will develop into healthy embryos. If they do, those healthy embryos are implanted in your uterus (or in the uterus of a surrogate), where they (again, hopefully) grow into future little bundles of joy. That is, of course, the end goal of this whole process.

2. It is a manipulation of the first half of your menstrual cycle.

Before I started the egg-freezing cycle, I was totally mystified. I suffered from a common misconception: I thought this would be a month-long process (partly because I had no idea of how my cycle actually worked). I knew there were shots involved, and almost-daily blood work, because friends of mine had gone through fertility treatments. But other than that, I had it all wrong. So now that I know better, let me try to demystify the process's (mercifully brief) timetable.

Fertility treatments are, put simply, manipulations of our menstrual cycle, designed to trick our bodies into doing two things. First, to produce a group of viable eggs that can be fertilized outside our bodies, and second, before embryo transfer, to begin preparing the uterine lining for pregnancy so that when the doctors transfer the embryo, your body is ready to accept it for implantation. For the purposes of egg freezing, let's just focus on the first part—because until you thaw your eggs, the second part does not yet apply.

Here is the simplest breakdown of what the average egg-freezing process looks like: First, it takes anywhere from ten to fourteen days, on average. (Mine was on the shorter side, because my ovaries reacted to the drugs very quickly.) Treatment begins on the second day of your period. On this day, you go to the doctor first thing in the morning so they can run your blood work and perform a transvaginal ultrasound. Yes, ladies, an ultrasound on the second, and usually heaviest, day of your period. Imagine a huge cylindrical object being moved around up there while that blood just keeps right on comin', and you will understand why this was probably one of the least pleasant parts of the process.

Yet this exam is very important, because it determines a few key things. The ultrasound gives the doctors a sense of how many follicles you tend to produce in a natural cycle. They do this on day two because this is before you have recruited that month's dominant follicle. The doctors are hoping to see several follicles—and, of course, the more the better.

The blood work, meanwhile, measures a few other things, most important, your FSH and AMH levels. The result of this test along with an AMH level previously measured helps the doctors determine the appropriate dosage for and regimen of your stimulation drugs. In general, you want your FSH to be no higher than 10 mIU/ml for stimulation. AMH levels vary and, you guessed it, decrease with age. So your normal levels will depend on how old you are. I was thirty-six, and I had an AMH reading of 2.45, which was well above average for my age. (I'm still patting myself on the back for that. Did I mention I like a little competition?) Just to give you some perspective, the average AMH level for a thirty-six-year-old is around 1.8; for a twenty-six-year-old, the average level is around 4. (The vast difference in these numbers just goes to show how significantly AMH declines in ten years—but I digress.) To sum up: the more follicles the better, while you hope for a low FSH level and a high level of AMH.

Let's move on and continue right on up to the egg retrieval. The second day of your menstrual cycle is when you begin administering all those injections we just talked about. Depending on your hormone levels at the beginning of your cycle, you might be given two or three different types of shots for the duration. In addition to your injections, you will also go to the doctor approximately every other day for further transvaginal ultrasounds, which allow the doctors to count and measure your follicles. They want them nice and big, and they want a good cohort of eggs. Blood is drawn each time you visit the clinic, in order to measure your hormone levels. This information helps the doctors adjust the dosage of drugs, if necessary. I would go in to the office in the morning, and that same afternoon, someone from my doctor's office would call and tell me what dosage of drugs to give myself for the next day or two.

When the doctors decide that your eggs are ripe enough for retrieval—this typically occurs around day eleven or twelve—they prepare you for your all-important trigger shot. As I mentioned, the timing of this shot is very important, because it is what causes the final maturation of your eggs and tells your body to get ready to ovulate, meaning your egg retrieval has to occur at just the right time so you do not ovulate before your doctor collects your eggs.

My cycle was much shorter than this. I took my trigger shot on day eight or nine, in the middle of the night—I remember setting an alarm so I would not miss the window. Then, about thirty-four hours later, I went in for my egg retrieval.

It definitely does not take an entire month, as I once thought. And most important, the thing to remember is this: if you are at a good fertility practice, they will hold your hand the whole time and tell you exactly what to do every step of the way. You will not need to get a degree in medicine just to get through the process.

3. Whatever you do, do not start this process at an Egg Freeze party.

On a chilly December evening, I rushed out of my office at around 5:30 p.m. and invited a couple of my lovely colleagues to come with me on a research excursion for my blog. (I did not want to go alone, and I thought they might learn something.) We piled into a cab in SoHo and traveled uptown in atrocious traffic. When we finally arrived, we headed into the warm, dark lobby of the ultra-swanky NoMad Hotel, located in the Flatiron District of Manhattan, where we were whisked into a room by an event coordinator. Within minutes, I was offered a cocktail. I started milling about with at least forty other women, all of us snacking on fancy hors d'oeuvres and surrounded by plush décor. My fellow attendees looked slightly bemused, not entirely sure of themselves. If I had to guess, I would say more than a few of these women were reconsidering their attendance at this somewhat surreal function (and I was starting to regret inviting my colleagues)—which was, if you have not already guessed, an Egg Freeze party, where perpetually smiling, hyper-friendly boosters of the procedure schmooze you, they hope, into preserving your fertility.

Buyer beware, though. Barb Collura, the CEO of RESOLVE—a nonprofit designed to help those suffering from infertility by offering them education, advice, and support—told me her sobering assessment of these parties: most of the information women receive about egg freezing is provided to them by people or organizations in a position to earn money if these women go forward with the procedure. Egg freezing is extremely lucrative for the clinics that provide the service, because it is not covered by insurance—meaning doctors can charge whatever the market will bear, without having to answer to insurance carriers. The service is also a boon for the adjacent industries that make egg freezing possible (such as cryogenic storage facilities, or suppliers of cryoprotectants). And as you may have guessed, the organizations that throw Egg Freeze parties also stand to gain enormously if they convince women to undergo the procedure. As of this writing, these gatherings are all the rage in New York, Los Angeles, and San Francisco, as well as in a few other burgeoning markets.

I use the word "market" intentionally. Because despite the way their organizers portray themselves, these parties are not educational sessions held out of the goodness of their hearts. These are savvy marketing ploys disguised as chic cocktail parties where a group of sunny "experts" supposedly gives you accurate and objective information. I am all for openness and honesty and discussing topics like these at cocktail parties—I think it is about time we stopped whispering about fertility and egg freezing, and if the best way for you to do that is while chatting over a mojito, so be it. But ladies, beware. When someone wants to sell you something, they are far less likely to be interested in maintaining objectivity or acknowledging the nuance of your particular situation. And when the subject at hand is your reproductive future—indeed, anything at all medical—that is problematic, to say the least.

One quick disclaimer: I am not inherently against earning money. I like capitalism. I think doctors should be fairly paid for their invaluable services. But as consumers, we have to be smart enough to decipher fact from fluffery, and when it comes to medicine, that can be hard to do for the average layperson on a *good* day—let alone once she is on her third glass of free chardonnay and is, in all likelihood, feeling vulnerable and scared about her reproductive potential. *That* is what makes these Egg Freeze parties potentially dangerous and somewhat predatory.

The event I attended at the NoMad—it was research for my blog, I swear!—was put on by EggBanxx, which again, is essentially a medical broker. The company invites various clinics from the area to participate in the event, and these clinics deploy their best-looking, most upbeat doctors to talk to the gathered crowd of hopeful future moms about the peace of mind that comes with egg freezing. Then a handful of smart, beautiful, articulate women who have undergone the procedure further rouse the crowd with their moving stories of empowerment and newfound peace of mind. Finally, guests leave with gift bags full of swag from the different clinics vying for their business and, if all goes to plan, call one of these clinics to set up a consultation appointment.

The company organizing the party negotiates discounts with these clinics (for the procedure only; the drugs still cost what they cost) in return for a certain volume of patients. If you, the patient, still cannot afford a cycle at the discounted rate, organizing company (EggBanxx, in this case) happily provides you with high-interest financing.

But let's try to keep an open mind for a moment. Gina Bartasi, CEO of Progyny, Inc., the company that owns EggBanxx and several other fertility-related starts-ups, argues (rightly) that these discounts and financing plans, however tasteless they may seem, are for many women the only way a cycle of egg freezing is financially possible. Bartasi pointed out to me that the prospect of insurance covering the procedure in the near future is not likely—so who else, she asked, is going to step into the fray and make egg freezing accessible to the women who might truly benefit from it? What is so wrong with giving these women the option?

Nothing at all. I take her point. Except that in these party-like sessions, the speakers can be downright disingenuous if it benefits them to spin the truth. For example, when I asked one doctor at the NoMad what he thought was the ideal age to freeze one's eggs, he told me anywhere between age thirty-five and thirty-seven. That is simply not true—it is not even *close* to being true, as we discussed earlier. But that doctor had read the crowd, and he knew most of the women in the room fell right into the age range he had specified. Medical reality or not, he clearly did not want to look us in the eye and tell us that the egg-freezing ship may have already sailed for us. Because who among us would set up an appointment and potentially shell out thousands after hearing that?

Just a quick side note: Currently, the average age at which women are freezing their eggs *is* around thirty-seven and a half—probably because that is when they actually start worrying about their chances of becoming a mom one day, and can finally afford to do something about it. It is certainly not, despite what that doctor told us, because thirty-seven and a half years old is the age at which you will generate the most eggs or have the highest chance of getting pregnant from those eggs. I find myself worrying about what sort of information these women are being fed. Are underhanded marketers simply telling women what they want to hear because it puts money in their pockets? After attending one of these events, you have to wonder.

Of course, some doctors want to help you split the difference and give a more realistic view of when it's best to freeze. They may tell you that the best age to freeze your eggs is between thirty-two and thirty-four, which is an age when you are more likely to be able to afford the procedure both financially and emotionally; when you will be more capable of spending the time and energy, and doing the future-focused thinking, that it will take to complete the process. But it is also an age at which your eggs are still likely to be plentiful and viable. (Me? I think you should have all the information when you are still able to create the most eggs possible.) Typically, doctors will not tell you that they do not believe your twenties are the ideal age to freeze, even though that's when your eggs are the healthiest (assuming you're a healthy, fertile woman), because at that age, they argue, you still have a high chance of having children naturally and so therefore, the risks do not outweigh the benefits—I say the patient should decide when the benefit outweighs the risk (after comprehensive research, conversations with a doctor, and a realistic view on when child bearing may actually be an option).

That said, the doctors I met at the NoMad were not entirely transparent about success rates, and I have heard from other attendees that a lot of magic math tends to float around at these things. One doctor told those in attendance that after three cycles of transfers of embryos created from your frozen eggs, you end up with an 85 to 90 percent take-home-baby rate. But that glosses over the fact that egg fertilization, embryo culture, and embryo transfers can be prohibitively expensive. In other words, the freezing is only half the battle. It would be like a slimy used car salesman selling you a car for ten grand—and then slyly mentioning that you will need to cough up another ten grand for the engine and wheels. If I'm using NYU numbers, one cycle of egg freezing is roughly between $10,000 and $15,000 (this includes drugs and things like anesthesia, which is not part of the cycle; again keep in mind that costs vary by city and clinic); an egg-thaw cycle (assuming you only thaw once) comes in at nearly $6,000, then the frozen embryo transfer cycle comes in at $4,000 (and keep in mind you can thaw and fertilize more than one egg at a time, so if your thawed eggs are successfully fertilized and turn into healthy embryos, the $6,000 is potentially a one-time fee, but you'll likely need three or more frozen embryo transfer cycles for a successful pregnancy). So, using the low end of the range, that's $10,000 for egg freezing, $6,000 for the thaw, and three times $4,000 for three frozen embryo transfer cycles, which adds up to $28,000, for an 85 to 90 percent chance of having a baby, ladies. Note that these costs don't account for other essentials like donor sperm (which can range anywhere from a few hundred bucks to thousands, depending on how much you need, how much information you have about the donor, etc.), important embryo testing, sperm cryopreservation, etc. If you were not paying close attention at that party—and do they really want you to, if they are handing you glasses of wine all night?—you might leave it thinking that one cycle of egg preservation, and nothing else, would result in heartening, nine-out-of-ten odds of pregnancy. But that is just not the whole story.

So here is the upshot: if you attend one of these parties, you join a captive, valuable (and more than a little vulnerable) audience.

4. The younger, the better.

Okay, now that I have gotten all that cynicism out of my system— sorry, not sorry—let's get back to just how astonishing it is that egg freezing is even a thing. Even if I never have a baby with one of my dear little hatchlings, the fact you can literally freeze your fertility in time still blows my mind. The general consensus amongst fertility doctors and embryologists is that egg freezing has made it so that eggs can be frozen indefinitely without damage (unless they are damaged during the thawing process). There is no expiration date! These eggs simply do not go bad.

But here is the thing: they need to be *good* in the first place. As we learned earlier, the success rate of eggs frozen before a woman is thirty-four is significantly higher than that of eggs frozen after that age. ("Success" being defined here as the ability to create a healthy baby.) That fact has real implications on any pregnancies that occur as a result of these frozen eggs. If you freeze your eggs at, say, age thirty-two, then implant an embryo made with those eggs at, say, forty years old, you will not need to undergo all the genetic tests that most women older than thirty-five do when they become pregnant naturally. (Good thing that, in this day and age, most forty-year-old women *are* in great shape. At thirty-eight, I feel better and healthier and more well balanced than I ever was in my late twenties or early thirties, because I have the means to take better care of myself).

So we have established that freezing younger is freezing smarter, right? Well, brace yourself for a catch-22. At the moment, most gynecologists actually make it a practice to *discourage* twenty-something women from freezing their eggs, because, they often say, these young women still have so many years to meet someone and have a baby naturally—so why undergo an expensive medical procedure that, like all medical procedures, carries a certain level of risk?

Kate has a (typically) wise theory about why gynecologists are hesitant to bring the procedure up in conversation. "Because for so long the technology of egg freezing was considered pioneering," she says, "a large chunk of the medical profession viewed it as a false promise. The tech wasn't good enough to make this procedure a real insurance policy, and the doctors feared that their patients would make life choices based on the wrong assumption. A lot of mainstream fertility doctors were saying, in its early days, 'Let's not talk about that.' The dialogue was like, 'Why freeze your eggs? Just go get pregnant now.'" For some doctors, that is still the best advice.

But while it still offers no guarantees, that faulty tech is now, of course, not so faulty. Still, while doctors, are of course, trained to consider risk versus benefit, sometimes they fail to discuss egg freezing for an even more objectionable reason. If you are, in their eyes, too young to be thinking about such things, they will likely tell you something like, "You still have plenty of time." If you happen to be twenty-two or twenty-six, they are probably right. If you are any older, you should take that advice with a major grain of salt.

Many, if not most, of the women of my tribe—well-educated, career-oriented urbanites attempting to balance life and work while still keeping an eye on the future—do not find Mr. Right nor get pregnant until well after their optimal childbearing years. Trust me on this, ladies. I know what you are thinking—because I used to think it too. You are thinking that surely things will be different for you, that you will be one of the lucky few who stumbles face-first into true and perfect love, and that babies will inevitably, effortlessly follow. But do not forget that in these next, most crucial years of your life, you will be busy working and living. Maybe too busy, in fact, to find the handsome husband, or to pencil in pregnancy and motherhood. Even if you do find the man, do not forget you might not get it right the first time—you might, in other words, marry the wrong man before you find the right one. (Hell, you might even marry a few wrong ones before you find the right one. It has been known to happen.) Whatever you wind up doing, just know that before long you will look up and be thirty-something or older, and you will find yourself thinking, *Where did the time go?*

I know I have said that to myself a million times. And I have heard many of my friends say it too. Such as Lauren, for example, who points out that this whole idea of "waiting too long" is bunk. Most of us are not "waiting" at all. "My mom was this pushy Jewish woman, the typical Jewish mom," she says. "I felt like I was a failure in her eyes. I wasn't producing a grandchild for her, wasn't in a committed relationship, which she reminded me of often. Yeah, do you think I don't know that? Do you think I'm doing it on purpose? She was like, 'You need to freeze your eggs.' I was really angry that she said that. I just felt like her comments were insensitive to my current life stage, and it's always like, when you're not dating someone, you don't need someone to point that out. 'Why aren't you married?' Well, I haven't found the right person!"

Kate told me something similar. "It irritates the hell out of me when people say in the popular discourse, in a magazine that's progressive and right-on in other respects, that women 'wait too long.' It's sloppy language. It's as if we're literally waiting. Like there aren't a million other things in our lives! I don't feel like I *waited*, I feel like I was trying to make it happen, but various factors not fully in my control determined the outcome. That wasn't me waiting. It's as though people think that if we simply put our minds to it we could make a baby happen, and that's just false." Hear, hear.

Let's break this down. You now know that eggs are far healthier when they are younger. You know (or are pretty sure) that you would prefer to have a baby when you are older or that you will not be able to afford a baby until then. You know things happen, and time slips through your fingers, and so you have to counter that with a little pragmatism and smart strategizing. With this information in mind, the question seems so simple: why should you not freeze your young eggs now, while they are still at their peak?

Of course, that is the logical question. But I do know that it is hard to think concretely about your future when you are just starting out in life. I mean, who has time to think about life's deep conundrums—*to parent or not to parent*, among them—when she can barely afford dinner? Another way to say this, care, once again, of dear Kate: "In your twenties kids are abstract. Maybe not for everyone, but they were for me."

In fact, when I asked my friends if they thought about their fertility when they were in their twenties, the answers were nearly the same across the board:

ALISON: "I did not think about it, not a bit."

AMELIA: "No, I definitely did not think about my fertility in my twenties."

LAUREN: "I rarely thought about it."

HEATHER: "Nope. People always said things like, 'You have so much time, you're so young.' I stopped hearing that after a while."

And, the answer I can definitely relate to:

VICTORIA: "Well, I thought about it in the sense of *not* getting pregnant."

However—and this is the really interesting part—when I asked my brilliant friends what they would tell their twenty-something selves now, their answers were staggering:

HEIDI: "The fertility conversation, the egg-freezing conversation, should just be normal when you are in your early twenties, so you can detach the *I hope I meet a guy* emotion from it. Scientifically, this is the best time. Who knows what is going to happen? But you should just do it. When you're younger you don't want to spend money on things like that, and you still have that hope. But if a bigger force can take away the money equation and make it more of a scientific narrative . . . I wish we were having *that* conversation."

VICTORIA: "I would definitely freeze my eggs sooner. When I went at thirty-four or thirty-five, my doctor basically said, 'You're already too late.' But that was when I did it, because I didn't have a choice. You should do it in your early twenties—though, of course, *nobody* in her early twenties does it, because it's too expensive and it can be intrusive, and also no one's gynecologist is even telling them it's an option! But just think of it this way: it's two weeks, and a certain amount of money that you can finance or borrow, and it saves you so much potential sadness down the line."

AMELIA: "Think about this *now*. It's crazy that there really isn't a dialogue about fertility prior to it being already a problem, or too late. When women are in their twenties—that's when it should be brought up with them. Getting the AMH test at twenty-seven or twenty-eight is such a minor box to check for a lot of peace of mind later in life. Because if you *are* losing fertility at a younger age than is assumed, how would you ever know that otherwise?"

Couldn't have said it better myself.

5. *It is eggspensive.*

A typical one-time cycle of egg freezing can cost anywhere from $8,000 to $10,000, depending on where you live and the clinic you go to. (I'm not including drug costs in this, which makes the numbers fuzzier because the drugs vary based on type, how much is needed, and whether or not insurance covers it—because some drugs are covered by some insurance companies). Even the "cheap" end of that spectrum, of course, is not a small amount of money to anyone except oligarchs and socialites—and it is a sum that is probably laughably out of reach for most women in their early or mid twenties. And, again, while some of the drugs are covered by a few insurance plans, insurance does not cover the egg-freeze cycle at all, anywhere, for any reason, except if you've been diagnosed with a disease that could damage your fertility (e.g., cancer). As of today, the healthcare industry has not caught up to, or has chosen not to catch up to, the fact that women are having to delay childbirth and, therefore, egg freezing is seen as entirely elective. It is entirely up to you to foot the bill.

But there is a silver lining to that part of things, at least. Some insurance policies—those that cover IVF, specifically—*will* cover some of the hormone injections associated with egg freezing, because they are associated with IVF. In other words, the stimulating shots you give yourself during the egg-freezing process are the same drugs you would give yourself if you were undergoing a cycle of IVF, so *if* (and that is a big *if*) your insurance covers IVF, those benefits might extend to egg freezing too.

Every policy is different, though. As I said, many of them require you to show a prior history of infertility before they will extend any fertility coverage at all. Which means that if you are a single woman who has not actively tried to get pregnant with fertility treatments, the drugs will not be covered at all, even if your plan does technically cover IVF. Try wrapping your head around that one.

But let's say your plan *does* cover the drugs. That is very, very good news, because the cost is wildly expensive. Personally, all in, I spent nearly $16,000 for my twenty-eight eggs to be frozen. That is around $571 per egg, which does not sound so bad. But when you consider that you typically need at least eight eggs to produce one live-born baby, that translates to about $4,568 per *half of* a *potential* child (half because the above calculation only accounts for freezing eggs not the thaw or the embryo transfer!).

How does that $16,000 break down? Here is the itemized list:

ITEMIZED COST OF MY EGG FREEZING + NATIONAL AVERAGES

- Hormone injections: approximately $5,000 (which was much more than I needed to spend because I ultimately didn't need all of the drugs!)

- Care and procedure: $9,200 (this includes your visits for blood work and ultrasounds every other day, plus the egg-retrieval surgery itself)

- Anesthesia: $1,200 (some clinics, like mine, charge for this separately rather than including it in the cost of the surgical procedure)

Of course, if all these steps do not ultimately yield enough viable eggs, you may be forced to repeat the cycle—which, obviously, doubles the cost. As I went through the egg-freezing process, I remember thinking to myself, *These eggs better be made of gold or at least result in some fantastic little human beings one day.*

Again, the above only accounts for part of the ability to preserve young eggs, so there is much more once you decide to actually try and get pregnant with your frozen eggs. You then need to consider the cost of thawing, fertilization, embryo culture, and transfer, in which your eggs are thawed and implanted in your body. Based on the costs at my clinic, this adds another nearly $6,000—and that is only for *one* transfer (not including drugs), which may or may not be successful. Because many people need multiple transfers, I should probably bank on a potential total of about $18,000 for three transfers (again, this doesn't account for the drug). Let's pause for a subtotal: In my case, it was nearly $16,000 for freezing the eggs (that does include the extras, like drugs and anesthesia), plus $16,000 to thaw, fertilize, and implant them. Let's assume that the drug costs will be comparable to my egg-freeze cycle, and I need three cycles: that adds about $12,000 (I'm *not* using the full $5,000 I paid for my egg-freeze drugs because I bought more than I needed). So, $16,000 (total for egg freezing) + $18,000 for three cycles of thawing and implanting + $12,000 for drugs. That comes out to $46,000. (Gulp.)

But wait, there's even *more!* The annual storage fee for my eggs was free for the first year—NYU threw that in as a little bonus (thanks, guys!)—but it cost around $1,000 per year after that. So let's assume I store my eggs for another five years before thawing. The storage fees might seem minimal—after all, what is another grand when you have just dropped sixteen of them?—but they are ongoing, and they add up.

So—drum roll, please—the final total for freezing my eggs, storing them for five years, thawing them, and then fertilizing and implanting them is (assuming I need three transfer cycles for success) . . . I am looking at around fifty grand.

To put that in perspective: before he or she is even born, I will have spent as much on my (potential, not-at-all-guaranteed) child as some parents spend on a year of college tuition. If ever I thaw my eggs and have the good fortune of having a baby from my very expensive, frozen eggs, allowance will certainly be out of the question, as I'll be starting in a hole.

But let me give the last word on this to Alison, who offers a little dose of perspective. "Well, let's think about the money for a second," she says. "A lot of people think, 'I don't have this much money! How am I supposed to do this?' But think of it this way: Do you lease a car? Do you have a home or an apartment? If you finance the procedure, your monthly payment can be $300 a month. I pay that for my car. We all pay several times that in rent or on a mortgage. Having children someday is so important that it is definitely worth it, at least to me."

6. You will need to embrace your inner hen!

For this procedure to truly be worth your time, money, and energy, you have to make sure to do one very important thing: lay a whole bunch of eggs! Doctors believe that, on average, you need eight frozen eggs to create one live born baby, and that is if you are on the younger side.

But as Drs. Druckenmiller and Noyes point out, that figure swells as you age. Here are a few rules of thumb for likely live births, broken down by age and number of mature eggs retrieved:

AT AGE TWENTY-FIVE to THIRTY-FOUR, you need

8 eggs, on average, to achieve live birth.

AT AGE THIRTY-FIVE to THIRTY-SEVEN, you need

10 eggs, on average, to achieve live birth.

AT AGE THIRTY-EIGHT to FORTY, you need

14 eggs, on average, to achieve live birth.

AT AGE FORTY-ONE to FORTY-TWO, you need

50 eggs, on average, to achieve live birth.

Yes, I know: those numbers are staggering. And even if you *do* manage to lay the right number of eggs, a child is not guaranteed. Nothing in this field is guaranteed, in fact—you might have noticed that already. This is in part because, unfortunately, doctors do not have a reliable way to evaluate the quality of our eggs until they are fertilized.

Obviously, I wanted to generate as many eggs as possible to increase my chances. But I am also a bit competitive by nature, and as such, managed to turn even *this* into a (friendly) contest. Lauren froze her eggs about six months before I froze mine. And her experience was a good one: she had a very successful procedure. In her blog entry, Lauren described how, one night, her boyfriend joked that she was "a good little laying hen" because she had laid thirty-six eggs. (That is a very respectable number. While there is no real "typical" number, because every woman is different, most women generate somewhere between five and fifteen eggs, depending on age, of course.) Of the thirty-six eggs Lauren laid, twenty-eight of them went on to be frozen. Not all eggs are fully mature at the time of collection.

Once I knew Lauren's magic number, I was determined to beat her at this whole egg-freezing thing. I would lay even more, I promised myself. I asked my doctors every day how many follicles I had grown, and couldn't they make me grow just a few more before the egg collection? When my numbers went up, and my follicles started to get "nice and juicy" (my doctor's words, not mine), I had the urge to high-five every doctor, nurse, or passerby in sight. I was obsessed with how many follicles I had, and how much they had grown, from day to day. The size is also important: in your natural cycle, one dominant follicle tends to emerge every moth, tending to be twenty-two to twenty-four millimeters in size. When you are freezing your eggs, you want to develops several follicles that are sixteen to twenty-two millimeters before retrieval.

In the end, Lauren and I froze the same number of eggs. I did not get to "win," sadly—but I did get to be a "good little laying hen," myself, and that is a big win in my book.

All joking aside, it can be devastating to lay too few eggs after expending all that time, money, and energy. Many women I know have gone through multiple cycles just to avoid that outcome. Sometimes doctors will actually stop a cycle or even recommend against starting it in the first place if they do not think they can stimulate the patient to produce a reasonable number of good eggs. They know that if you cannot yield enough mature eggs, the cost of the procedure may wind up outweighing any benefit you might derive from it. Your doctor can help determine if you will react well to the shots and produce the number of eggs needed by measuring your FSH and AMH levels; these are typical tests that any doctor will run prior to starting a cycle.

Funnily enough, if I laid thirty-four eggs every month, I would actually be more productive than the average commercial laying hen, which lays about 275 eggs per year. Lucky for me, I only had to do it for *one* month—and that was plenty, because when you are gearing up for egg retrieval, you do begin to feel like little more than an incubator. For that one cycle, your body's sole focus is to produce as many eggs as possible.

Now we get to the part where I tell you why this whole laying hen concept is so important for you to know in advance. There are consequences to treating your body this way—to making it generate something at a rate and volume that is, in a word, unnatural. Going big on egg production means, in my experience, going a little nuts. My doctor referred to mine as "lunatic ovaries" at one point. Keep in mind that in a typical month, *one* follicle matures. I had *thirty-four* of them crowding my ovaries, and said ovaries were really not happy about it. They were sore and full, and anything that sore and full is awfully distracting. (In fact, my ovaries were angrier with me than most—I developed what is known as ovarian hyperstimulation syndrome, which we will get to later.) My ovaries also swelled considerably. I do not exaggerate when I say that I looked five months pregnant by the end of my cycle. In fact, my friend Stella actually *was* five months pregnant at the time, and our tummies looked identical.

Worst of all, when your ovaries are stimulated, they demand stillness. Your doctors absolutely, positively do not want you exercising, lifting, twisting, or anything else even vaguely resembling movement or activity. I thought I could exercise for the first few days of the cycle but was told to stop right away—it turns out you can seriously hurt yourself if your ovaries become twisted and the blood supply gets tangled. (Yes, that can actually happen.) And you cannot start exercising again until your ovaries are back to their normal size, which sometimes does not happen for a couple weeks after the egg-retrieval procedure.

The point is, there will be a portion of your egg-freezing journey during which you will become a mere vessel for your tiny, precious, massively expensive cargo—and the psychological and physical effects of that part of the process may be significant.

And speaking of psychological changes . . .

7. *The hormones may make you, well, a tad hormonal.*

To grow all these follicles I just mentioned, one needs drugs. Lots and lots of drugs. These drugs enter your body in the form of injections. Lots and lots of injections, (for me, it was a total of 18 self-administered shots in just under two weeks). The result is that your ovaries become prolific egg factories—and, oh yeah, you also might become a weepy, enraged mess.

But let's back up a moment and discuss the injections and hormones themselves. The injections are probably the most grueling part of the egg-freezing process, because they have to be administered multiple times a day, for several days—and for most of us, at least, puncturing our own skin on a regular basis is not exactly a lifelong dream. Okay, I am being snarky; they really are not that bad. But they are frequent, which takes commitment, and like every other aspect of this undertaking, they are pricey.

Just before the egg-freezing cycle begins, you need to order a big batch of the drugs from your pharmacy. Here is an incredibly important tip: do not order the full prescription all at once! Depending on how well and rapidly you stimulate your ovaries, you may not need every last drop of that medication. In fact, it has been a year since I froze my eggs, and I still have about $3,000 worth of Follistim sitting in my fridge. (Turns out you cannot return what you do not use, and it is illegal to sell it. If only I had known I would be such a quick, efficient layer of eggs!)

The evening my drugs arrived—they were delivered from the pharmacy, carefully packaged and chilled—that aforementioned fridge was filled to the brim with champagne, wine, and leftovers. (Don't judge, I like to keep a little bubbly and vino around, just in case. . . .) In fact, I struggled to make room for the ten boxes of Follistim. I remember thinking my fridge contained just what every modern bachelorette's should: booze, takeout, and thousands of dollars worth of hormone injections.

I was so scared of the shots, I have to admit. Turns out, they were the easiest part of the whole process. First of all, they were far less painful than I imagined they would be. In fact, the injections really do not hurt at all. The needles are tiny, which helps. You just lift up a bit of skin and quickly stick yourself. I would grab a small fold slightly below and to the side of my belly button, moving the injection site around each day to avoid bruising or soreness. While some women opt to engage a nurse to come over and give them their injections, I did not think it was necessary. Because it is just skin you are puncturing, not muscle, it is actually pretty easy—kind of like sticking a needle in butter, in fact.

But what *are* these crazy-making substances you will be asked to pump into your body multiple times a day? Let's go down the list:

Gonadotropins are hormones used to stimulate the follicles that grow eggs during the stimulation phase of the egg-freezing cycle. Brands you might be prescribed include Follistim, Gonal-F, and Menopure. These hormones will likely comprise the bulk of your medication during this process, because stimulating follicle development is the most important thing you need to accomplish (especially if you are trying to out-hen your friends). You will give yourself up to two shots of this stuff each day, though dosing will depend on your personal follicle count and hormone levels at the beginning of the cycle and throughout the stimulation phase. This stuff helps you go from a normal ovulator to a laying hen.

Some gonadotropins, like the one I used, come in a pen-like syringe with a small needle extending from one end; these types also feature a stupid-proof mechanism to make sure you accurately measure out how much to give yourself. (They look just like EpiPens, if you have ever seen one of those.) The hardest part is getting the little vial of medicine into the pen (and that is not that hard at all, really—you may just feel a bit clumsy at first). Other brands require setting up a little mini-lab in your kitchen to mix various powders and liquids. Heather wound up with this kind of drug—and while preparing her doses was slightly more complicated than me taking the cap off my Follistim pen, the process did make us feel like accomplished scientists. Whether you wind up with the pen or the powders depends on your doctor's recommendation; some of the drugs fit different situations and patients better than others.

Next up are GnRH agonists and antagonists, which prevent spontaneous—aka natural—ovulation. While the gonadotropins help you make as many follicles with eggs in them as possible, these guys ensure that you don't lose all those eggs by ovulating before the egg retrieval, which would be bad. If you dropped your eggs before they could be collected, you'd have to start all over. Examples of this class of medication include buserelin, leuprorelin, nafarelin, and triptorelin.

Yes, the GnRH agonist and antagonist is another round of shots. Which one you are administered depends on which treatment protocol your doctor prescribes. The GnRH agonists have been around longer and were used more frequently in the 90s and early 2000s. This ovulation stopper is usually started a week prior to the treatment month and continues until two days before the egg retrieval. The most common one used in the U.S. is leuprolide acetate.

GnRH antagonists work by preventing natural ovulation by preventing the mid-cycle hormonal surge of luteinizing hormone

(LH). Typically, these hormones are given beginning in the middle of the stimulation phase of treatment, after gonadotropins have begun their stimulation work but before the ovulation trigger shot. Examples of this class of medication include Ganirelix and Cetrotide. This is the natural-ovulation preventer I was told to take. In total, I was prescribed three single-dose, pre-mixed injections of GnRH antagonist—ones where I just tossed the entire syringe when finished. Best of all, this was another simple shot with a super-thin needle that could be injected in skin rather than muscle. Easy.

Last, about thirty-four hours prior to the egg retrieval, a trigger shot is given (and your doctors are *not* kidding around with that timing—you need to give yourself the injection within ten minutes of whatever time your doctor tells you. That shot assists in the final maturation process of the eggs, by causing them to undergo a reproductive division called meiosis, and also causes the mature eggs to be released from the follicles. For this reason, the shot needs to be timed precisely with egg collection so you don't end up ovulating away your hard-earned eggs. The trigger shot most often consists of hCG but may include a combination of hCG plus a GnRH agonist, or simply a GnRH agonist alone.

In most cases, only one trigger shot is needed, hCG. But women who are at risk of ovarian hyperstimulation syndrome—like me, for instance—most often get a combination of these shots, to minimize the risk of their ovaries going crazy. So on Super Bowl Sunday 2015, while most people were overdosing on beer and buffalo wings, I was preparing for my "harvest," or retrieval, by giving myself these two trigger shots at around midnight. These too were premixed for me by the pharmacy, which they waited to do—as is typical—until the day I needed it.

Now I come to the part about how pumping your body full of hormones might—to put it mildly—alter your mood. The gist is this: You cannot raise your follicle count without also raising your estrogen levels, which are tied to the number of follicles being produced.

In a normal cycle, your one dominant follicle secretes estrogen. When you go through an egg-freezing cycle, the goal is to generate more follicles than just one—which means that once the group of eggs all starts secreting in concert, your estrogen levels will be much, much higher than usual.

Mine, in fact, shot straight through the roof. When I started my cycle, my estrogen level was 45. A couple days and a few shots later, it climbed to 458, then, in another forty-eight hours, to 987. Six days in, I was clocking in at more than 2,000, and at the end of the cycle, I was around 4,000. *That is a lot.* I had at least one meltdown per day, usually in the evening, as I was injecting my last shot. I would cry and feel sorry for myself and ask questions like "What am I doing laying eggs when I should be having babies?" One minute I felt tired and hazy, while at other moments I felt energized, clearer than I had felt in a long time. (I also had not gone so long without alcohol in ages, so that could have been a contributing factor.) Sometimes I felt strange, almost superhuman. But no matter what I felt, I was always *very* emotional—roughly two seconds from tears at all times. It may have been partially about the huge significance of what I was doing—this was a big choice, and it meant, and still means, a lot to me—but I also think my estrogen levels were just making me insane. For all our talk about not blaming our bad behavior on hormones, I think if I had killed someone, a judge would have found me not guilty by reason of insanity.

The worst part of the hellish hormone experience was still to come, however. After having been hopped up on these drugs for eight days, I crashed. When I stopped the injections and my estrogen levels began to drop back to normal, I developed a migraine that did not quit—and it lasted for nearly a week! All the prescription drugs and acupuncture and sleep in the world did nothing to quell the pain. I just had to soldier through it until my body readjusted to human levels of estrogen. It definitely wasn't pleasant, but it was for a good cause. And I assure you I would do it again in a heartbeat, insanity, migraine, and all.

8. Egg retrieval is no walk in the park— it is an invasive procedure.

The last step of the oocyte cryopreservation process is egg retrieval. There is often a misconception that egg retrieval is some kind of breezy in-and-out proposition, like a teeth cleaning or pap smear. That is just not the case. It is not a major operation—you are only out for about fifteen minutes—but it is still invasive. It involves sticking a long needle through the vagina into the ovaries, then sucking the eggs out of the follicles with that needle. You should know that going into this process.

I mention that because I have heard stories of women who had to have the retrieval done while awake—some because they forgot they were not supposed to eat or drink for twelve hours before the procedure, as is standard practice before receiving anesthesia (which is always a risk in and of itself). Now, it is a simple and fast enough procedure that it *can* be done while you are awake, but I would not recommend it, especially if you are squeamish, like me. I mean, why experience a second of pain that you do not have to?

Speaking of not eating beforehand, I—having actually followed the rules—hadn't had a single bite in the twelve hours before my surgery. So naturally, I went into the whole thing quite "hangry." My mom had been with me throughout the whole process, shots and all, but having her around for this part was most important of all. You need someone to bring you home from the procedure, because you will be quite out of it. We went to NYU Langone Medical Center at ten in the morning—precise timing is everything, as I said—and I suited up into a dressing gown and a little shower cap–like hat to cover my hair. A lovely British nurse with a calming sense of humor made small talk as she took me to get my vitals checked. I remember her making a comment about how men have no idea about the things we women have to go through—that they are rarely subjected to such intrusive procedures near their reproductive body parts, and certainly never as an elective or conscious decision! She gave me some trashy magazines to read while I waited, then finally escorted me into the operating room.

Here is something I did not expect: the operating room was abuzz. I could not believe how many doctors and nurses were present for a procedure that was supposedly quick and simple. In any case, I climbed up onto the operating table to find warm, heated blankets waiting for me. Another soothing nurse rubbed my hands and told me it would be okay. The anesthesiologist told me I was about to have the best nap of my life. It all felt far more like a spa than a clinic. If not for the bright lights and the beeping machines, I would have thought I was going in for a body scrub. And then I was asleep.

Up to that point, my egg-freezing process had been so easy. My ovaries had cooperated, doing just what they were supposed to do. My jacked-up hormone levels had actually made me feel pretty good a lot of the time (if insanely emotional). The shots were so easy I almost enjoyed doing them. All in all, the whole experience had been straightforward, even pleasant.

That was all about to change.

9. All good things have a little risk attached.

It does not take a genius to recognize the pattern: when your ovaries are overachievers, there are consequences. Little did I know I would suffer a complication. But please do not think my story is normal, or that it will necessarily happen to you.

I woke up from the egg-retrieval procedure with the most intense cramps I had ever felt; it was as though my ovaries were screaming at me for what I had just put them through. Despite the pain, my first words (presumably they were quite slurred) were, "How many eggs did I get?" They told me thirty-four. Thirty-four! Had I not been severely dazed and also in mortal agony, I might have done a victory lap.

The doctors gave me painkillers through the IV, which was a relief—except that I had a weird reaction to them. My blood pressure became erratic, going from super low to super high, which was especially strange given that I have *amazing* blood pressure (yes, that is another thing I take pride in!). I watched as other patients came into and went out of recovery, spending about forty-five minutes there, total. Meanwhile, I was stuck in the room for several hours. So I began to panic. Yes, I had been an awesome laying hen, but I was clearly not so good at this part. Competitive little thing that I am, I was—even in the midst of my terror—somewhat annoyed that all the other women seemed to handle this part like it was nothing, looking like they had just had a massage and were about to go have their tea in the lounge. To make myself feel better, I told myself they had probably laid way fewer eggs than I had. What a bunch of losers. (Kidding, kidding.)

Now, not being a doctor, I cannot say for sure that my experience in the recovery room had anything to do with ovarian hyperstimulation syndrome—characterized by swollen, painful ovaries, thanks to the jillion eggs within them—or if I just had a bad reaction to the drugs. But whatever caused my extended stay in that room, it was a sign of things to come. My recovery took weeks. I struggled, day after day. While many women go back to work right after the procedure (even though that is not recommended, because the anesthesia remains in your system even after you wake up, causing drowsiness), I was out of commission for a week, and had to be monitored the entire time.

The symptoms of hyperstimulation can include rapid weight gain, abdominal pain, shortness of breath, and swelling in the abdomen—so much so that you look like you are pregnant. (I was already quite swollen during the harvest, and became even more so after the retrieval.) I had all those symptoms. My mom had to run out and buy a scale after my procedure, because the nurses told me to weigh myself the next morning (I did not own a scale before all of this; I don't believe in them!). If I gained more than four or five pounds—of water weight, not to worry—I was to come in immediately. Sure enough, I put on six pounds overnight! It felt hard to breathe. I was extremely uncomfortable. It became so painful I found it difficult to move.

If someone suffering from ovarian hyperstimulation syndrome accumulates enough fluid, she may actually need to have that fluid drained. Mine never got that bad, but poor Lauren was not so lucky. She is a tiny person—I assume her ovaries are tiny too—so producing thirty-four eggs put her girls into such severe hyperstimulation that she actually had to be admitted to the hospital, where the excess fluid in her body was drained with a needle. It did not sound fun at all. "That was really painful," Lauren says. "It felt like I couldn't breathe or sleep, they had swollen so badly. It was scary."

It was downright awful contending with all these symptoms on top of recovering from the procedure itself and the tail end of a crazy estrogen roller coaster. But this was a means to an end—part of a process I knew I had to undertake. Anything worth having involves a little risk. And even if I had known my ovaries would mutiny after my egg-collection procedure, I still would have done it. While there are no guarantees to be found in the world of egg freezing, I do not ever want to be the sort of person who shies away from going after what she truly wants just because she is afraid of taking a risk.

10. You may still be baby crazy afterward.

The reality is that this section will not apply to you if you freeze your eggs before you are ready to actually become a mother. These days, many women, including myself, freeze their eggs as a reaction to a relationship gone wrong, or things not turning out the way they had planned. But if you freeze as an objective, preemptive option well before you hear your biological clock ticking, you can probably bypass this section entirely.

While I am indeed the happy owner (or should I say mom?) of twenty-eight little hatchlings, all safely (and coldly) stored somewhere in Manhattan, the fact is my ovaries still hurt every time

I see a baby. And in a perfect world, I would still get what I have always wanted: career + husband/partner + baby. But I am certainly more open to the possibility of doing the whole baby thing on my own than I ever was, and that openness has come about with time and age—not, as you might think, from freezing my eggs.

Which is to say that freezing your eggs will not necessarily quell your yearning for a child. After successfully completing the oocyte cryopreservation process, I remember thinking, *Congratulations, you have . . . twenty-eight frozen eggs!* While it felt good to know I had taken some action, suspending my thirty-six-year-old eggs in time, there were moments when I felt that I should have just taken the next step and tried a round of IUI with donor sperm.

Each woman has a different experience with freezing her eggs. My experience was influenced largely by the fact that not long before I went through the process, I had been trying to start a family with my ex. For me, it was an emotional journey. For other women, it may simply be a medical procedure that provides a bit of insurance, a way to get back to life without the nagging voice that says time is running out. For younger women, who are perhaps not yet baby desperate, egg freezing may simply be a smart, proactive procedure. It is different for everyone.

I think it is worth mentioning that this procedure may not be the emotional or psychological silver bullet you are looking for. For me, the biggest epiphany was that while I was glad I froze my eggs, at the time, I still wanted a baby just as much as I did before the freeze. Freezing my eggs did not immediately put my maternal urges on hold, and it did not immediately stop my biological clock from screaming at me every time I bounced a friend's baby on my knee or passed a stroller in the park. Perhaps that was because I froze my eggs soon after my failed marriage and failed attempts at getting pregnant. But what it has done is give me some time and space, to figure out what I'm going to do, and how I'm going to do it; it has given me the chance to really evaluate if I want a child on my own, or if I want one only with a partner, or if I want one at all. And while not everyone goes through this process under the emotional circumstances I did (in fact, like I said earlier, if you are doing this in your twenties, before the baby urges have kicked in, this may be irrelevant to you), I think it is important to know that you may not immediately be soothed simply by the action of having frozen your eggs.

11. Sometimes you do not get to have your eggs and hatch them too.

While I have zero regrets about taking control of my fertility future (or at least feeling as though I have taken control, which is almost as good), there is no guarantee that having done so will someday result in my having a baby of my own. In fact, critics of egg freezing are quick to point out its low success rates. But those statistics can be misleading— particularly because many frozen eggs have not yet been thawed, fertilized, and implanted. In other words, it may just be too soon to say.

But there are some statistics that are available when we look at the data. Back to Drs. Druckenmiller and Noyes, who offer the following figures:

SUCCESS RATES FOR THAWED EGGS

- Percentage of all frozen eggs that survive thaw: around 80 percent

- Percentage of all surviving eggs that fertilize properly: around 70 percent

- Percentage of all fertilized eggs that make it to blastocyst (a structure in early embryonic development): around 35–40 percent

The point is, only 25 percent of the eggs you have frozen will eventually become a blastocyst that will be used for transfer, and not all of these blastocysts will be "good-quality." In unfortunate cases, it is possible that none of the frozen eggs will develop into an implantable embryo or that none of the implanted embryos will develop into a live-born baby.

This is heartbreaking, I know. But it is also possible that your eggs will go unused because you simply never get around to using them. While the knowledge that I have twenty-eight hatchlings safely stored away for some future day has made me feel better about my reproductive future, whether or not I will ever have a baby with those eggs is still unclear, just as it is for many other women who have frozen their eggs.

12. Fertilization does not guarantee success.

We have talked a lot about the process of growing your eggs and having them retrieved, but we have not spoken much yet about how you will *store* those eggs. When it comes to how you preserve them, you have three options:

1. Freeze them solo.
2. Fertilize your eggs with sperm, then freeze them as embryos.
3. Opt for the combo platter, freezing some eggs unfertilized and some as embryos.

There are two schools of thought on this decision. One says that frozen embryos have a higher likelihood of making it to a live birth. The other says that the difference in success rates is clinically insignificant. So if you are a single woman who wants the opportunity to thaw those eggs with someone in the future, what is the better option? That decision comes down to you and your preferences—how you expect your future to shape up, how you feel about each option, and what your doctor advises.

Here is a bit of necessary context. One study showed that women have an 89 percent chance of making it to the transfer stage—i.e., the part of the process in which the embryo is implanted in your uterus—with a frozen egg, versus a 93 percent chance of making it to transfer with a frozen embryo. That 4 percent difference is largely due to the fact that some eggs are damaged in the freezing or thawing process; this risk appears less pronounced for embryos. Because oocytes are much more watery than embryos—they are 80 percent water— freezing them carries a higher likelihood of crystallization.

Personally, that 4 percent difference was okay with me. Because I was still holding out hope that I would meet the right person someday, I was not ready to commit to a donor's genetic material just yet. (Imagine if I fell in love and the gentleman and I decided to have a baby—but all I had on hand were eggs prefertilized by a sperm donor. Awkward.) In addition, in my case, Dr. Noyes advised me not to fertilize. She pointed out that the difference in success rates was about a 3:2 ratio, meaning 3 eggs equaled 2 embryos, and so someone with a good response to the fertility medication (like me) probably didn't need to make that compromise. Having said that, she did say that one of the advantages of frozen embryos (versus unfertilized eggs) is knowing they did fertilize, one step further on the road to implantation. If your eggs are not great at the time of retrieval, then it really does not matter if you fertilize ten right after the egg retrieval, or years down the road. The eggs are what they are.

Let me break down the math using my batch of twenty-eight eggs as an example.

THE BREAKDOWN:
HOW MANY EGGS DOES IT TAKE TO MAKE A BABY?

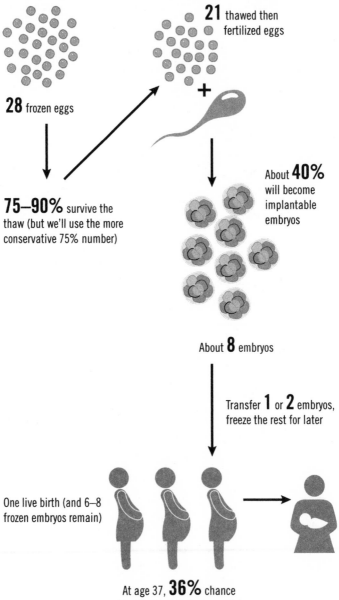

21 thawed then fertilized eggs

28 frozen eggs

75–90% survive the thaw (but we'll use the more conservative 75% number)

About **40%** will become implantable embryos

About **8** embryos

Transfer **1** or **2** embryos, freeze the rest for later

One live birth (and 6–8 frozen embryos remain)

At age 37, **36%** chance that the first embryo results in a live birth. It will probably take three transfers to work.

The gist is this: I have frozen twenty-eight eggs; 75 to 90 percent of those eggs will survive the thaw. (Yes, that is quite a wide range, which is because the numbers vary depending on whom you ask, how good the batch of eggs is, and how good the lab freezing your eggs is, at both freezing and thawing. EggBanxx, for example, quotes a 90 percent survival rate, which, of course, may be a bit self-serving and should be taken with a *big* grain of salt; more conservative clinics quote 75 percent survival rates. Dr. Druckenmiller says there is no one number, and that different embryologists obtain different survival rates.) Let's go with the 75 percent rate for the sake of argument. If I thaw twenty-eight eggs, I will likely be left with twenty-one to fertilize. Of these, about 40 percent will become implantable embryos. So at this stage, I will be left with about eight embryos to transfer. At NYU Langone Medical Center, my clinic, doctors normally only transfer one to two embryos into the uterus at a time (this decreases the likelihood of producing multiple embryos like twins or triplets, which make for many more risks during pregnancy). This means I would have one to two blastocysts transferred, while the rest would be frozen. Once the embryos are transferred, at my age there is about a 30 to 36 percent chance of the embryos making it to a live birth. (Again, that figure would be approximately the same whether the embryos being transferred were fresh or frozen.) So by virtue of simple math, it is likely I would need to go through three rounds of IVF transfers for a successful outcome. But even if I had to do three rounds, I would still be left with five blastocysts in the deep freeze, giving me a high chance of having a second child from the same batch of eggs.

But before you decide what is right for you, there are a few more factors to consider. First up: If you are single and want to fertilize your eggs before freezing them, you will need to be ready to go on a serious genetic shopping trip. There is a whole world of sperm banks out there, and they are set up for you to be able to browse through dozens upon dozens of men, much like you would on an online dating site. There are, of course, a few key differences between a sperm donor site and a dating platform, though: the former offers a bit more information than you get on Match.com, which does not usually reveal a potential date's health records, IQ, or STD status.

A word to the wise: It can be incredibly overwhelming to browse through pages and pages of potential genetic donors. When I considered single motherhood via the use of donor sperm, I came up with a strategy. At first, I decided I would use sperm from a man who resembled the sort of guy I would date; I tend to go for my physical opposite—dark and broody to my blonde and sunny. I have also always had this notion that children from couples who look dissimilar are cuter than the kids born of two blond or brown-haired parents. Of course, I have no empirical evidence for this, but that was my bias as I browsed the digital pages of California Cryobank. This was when I had another epiphany: *What if this child ends up looking nothing like me, and bears a very strong resemblance to a stranger?* Could I deal with strangers commenting on how Johnny or Janie must *really* take after his or her father? While I plan to be honest about my route to parenthood, whichever route it may turn out to be, I'm not sure I want to reveal the source of my genetic material during playground small talk. I also do not want my kid to deal with a constant reminder that he or she does not know his or her dad. Single parenthood will be complicated enough, so why add another potential layer of discomfort? So new strategy, should I go the single mom route: pick someone who looks just like me!

Of course, going the sperm donor route is not a draining experience for everyone. Victoria, who had her bouncy baby boy as a single woman via IUI, found the whole process to be easy as pie. "It was a very simple process—it's a lot easier to pick than you might think, provided you know what you want. Or at least it was for me, because I knew exactly what I wanted: a man who wasn't short and who was an academic and who was healthy, and I wanted it to be an anonymous donation. I wanted him to be Jewish, because I'm Jewish. And once you start to narrow down the field based on your criteria, the list gets fairly short. I think I worried about it a lot less than everyone else. I was decisive: *I'll take him.* Then it was done, and that was that."

Another thing to consider if you are leaning toward fertilizing before freezing: are you ready to make that commitment? If you are freezing because you are still looking, what happens if, after you have fertilized your eggs with some handsome stranger's swimmers, you do actually meet someone? Your frozen material will now be tied up with another man's genes.

Remember, however: the younger you are, the less this is an issue. If you are not comfortable with that 4 percent difference and are in your mid twenties, go ahead and fertilize away. You still have around ten good years—maybe more—to get pregnant naturally. But the later you freeze in life, the more likely it is that you will actually need those eggs. So bear that in mind.

13. Sometimes you will choose not to hatch them.

Perhaps this statement startles or surprises you. WTF, you may be thinking. *We just talked about how involved and emotional and expensive this whole undertaking can be! You really think I'm going to go through all that only to abandon my hatchlings in the deep freeze?*

Well, here is the thing with fertility—and with life in general: Things happen. Things you never expected to happen, more specifically. What sort of things? You might, for example, hit the jackpot and get pregnant naturally, rendering those frozen eggs irrelevant. You might get pregnant using IVF and one of your more recently hatched, non-frozen eggs. (If that sounds insane to you, keep reading; we will get to that in a moment.) You might experience a change of heart and find that having children is no longer the burning priority it once was for you. (Yes, this can happen. You might decide your career or creative pursuit or wanderlust or child-averse boyfriend is simply more important to you than being a mom. People are allowed to change their minds, and they often do.) You might fall in love with someone who already has children and discover that being a stepmom is just as fulfilling for you as being a mom-mom. You might look deep within and realize you feel a moral and spiritual calling to adopt. Hell, you might wake up one morning and discover a baby on your doorstep. You just never know. Life is wildly, thrillingly, and constantly unpredictable. Things happen—and you simply cannot predict which things will happen to you. (And isn't that a good thing? Life would get awfully boring otherwise.) And as a result of whatever wild stuff goes down in this life of yours, you may find that your desire to thaw those frozen eggs either wanes or disappears.

According to the Society for Assisted Reproductive Technology, roughly 9,000 women froze their eggs between 2009 and 2013 (the most recent year for which figures are available). The number of women undergoing the procedure skyrocketed after 2012, which was the year the "experimental" label was removed from the process and egg freezing became an elective procedure. Yet many of these frozen eggs are currently sitting in cryogenic storage units across the country. Each year since 2009, the gap between eggs frozen and eggs thawed has widened considerably. Drs. Druckenmiller and Noyes report that at NYU, there is a three-year lag, on average, between when a woman freezes her eggs and when she returns to thaw them. While research into the long-term viability of eggs and embryos is still scant—the technology just has not been widely available long enough to undertake such studies—some available research indicates that eggs and embryos remain viable after being frozen for five years; doctors and researchers are not yet certain about viability after periods longer than that. But the point is, many of these eggs are going unthawed. And many may never be thawed or used at all.

When I inquired, tentatively, about making use of my frozen eggs and pursuing fertility treatments alone about a year after what my brothers like to call my "big freeze," my doctor recommended that I first start with IUI (using donor sperm), then move up to IVF using fresh eggs rather than my frozen ones. This surprised me. But my doctor reminded me that those frozen eggs are like precious diamonds, not to be touched until I need them—in other words, when I am no longer able to produce healthy eggs on my own. And since I had been able to produce a great many good-looking eggs (we will not know for sure how good they actually are until we try to fertilize them; research on the genetic testing of unfertilized eggs is still— forgive the pun—in its infancy), my doctor felt I should try to use a fresh egg for my IVF, and hang on to the frozen ones for a rainy day.

But what if that rainy day never comes? What does one *do* with her unused eggs? This is actually among the first questions your clinic will ask you before you set off on your egg-freezing journey: "What would you like to do with any eggs that do not wind up hatching?" (My words, not theirs.) Your options are fairly limited: donate them to science, give them to some deserving woman or couple to help them create a baby, or discard them. But the emotional reaction you experience when your eggs go unused is sometimes far less straightforward.

Personally, I am not, at present, emotionally attached to my little frozen eggs in the same way I might be if they were embryos. To me, at the current moment, they are simply cells developed under severely hormonal circumstances, then surgically removed from my body; they do not, in and of themselves, have the capacity to create a life. But I am also aware that they represent hope—hope that I will one day have babies, even if that does not happen the old-fashioned way. And because of this, I am not sure how I might feel if I never used those eggs.

I have friends who are fellow freezers. Most of them say they will not know how they will feel about not using their eggs until they know *why* they are not using them—in other words, their emotional response will depend on their circumstances.

Alison says she doesn't expect to have a huge emotional investment in her unused eggs, but she would love for them to help someone else. "Throughout the process, I sat in that waiting room surrounded by so many women and couples shelling out so much money and praying with everything they had for a miracle," she says. "If I can give them that, why wouldn't I? Because it would be weird to know that I might have kids out there who are half mine? Yeah, that doesn't bother me; I don't stress too much about it. And if I do wind up using any of these golden eggs, I will happily gift any extras to a well-deserving friend or a total stranger. The world needs a little more Alison in it anyway."

Amelia would also donate her frozen eggs if she did not need to use them herself. "From what my doctor has said, I should have a good chance of getting pregnant on my own if I try in the next few years," she says. "Which means that these eggs could just be in reserve if I wanted to have a second or third child somewhere down the road. Which, at thirty-five, seems like a bit much. But if I'm not successful at getting pregnant on my own, I do have this option. I also have two sisters that are younger, and I think if they couldn't get pregnant, I would want them to have them. We're fairly close, so that has crossed my mind. But the truth is, of course, that I don't know what's going to happen to the eggs."

Heidi takes a (characteristically) firm position on the subject. "Well, I'm not using a lot of my eggs right now, right? In my natural cycle, a lot of eggs are being thrown out. I really don't feel an emotional attachment to the eggs. I don't. I don't think anyone would want them, because I was older when I froze them. I mean, obviously I've got some amazing genetic material. But if I still feel the same way I do now at, say, forty-two—I don't know why forty-two is the threshold in my mind; it just is—and someone wanted them, I'd have no problem giving them away."

Similarly, Victoria does not feel it would be difficult to donate her unused eggs. This question is more top of mind for her because, being a new mother to a young son, she is not sure she wants to have more children. "My mother is dead against my having more," she says. "What's that old saying? 'One child is a luxury, two is a liability?' I don't know, honestly. It's too early to know. I have the eggs, the sperm. . . . I don't have the embryos, but they could easily be created. I've been very lucky that my child is a delightful, delicious little boy, but apparently they aren't all like that, I've been told. The doctors tell you not to have another child for eighteen months, so maybe when it's closer to that time I'll give it more thought. But I think I would donate them. I would not feel conflicted about that, if it helped someone. If I can help someone, I want to."

Heather thought she had no attachment to her eggs—but then one month her bill for storing them was late, and she realized she felt more protective of them than she thought. "I panicked," she says, "because I didn't want them to think I wasn't going to pay and then toss them. If a hurricane was to hit and the eggs were destroyed, it would be hard for me to know that I can't get them back. If I wasn't able to make the decision about their fate, I'd be really upset about that."

I suppose I look at this question in roughly the same way—how I feel about not using my eggs will depend on the reason *why* I do not use them. If I make the decision to donate those eggs to science because I have a baby through other means, I do not think I will feel a single pang about letting them go. In fact, I believe I will feel *good* about contributing what I can to an area of medicine that needs more and continued research. If I fulfill the dream of becoming a mom without using those frozen eggs, I suspect they will become, to me, just meaningless cells taken from my body; I will have no more emotional attachment to them than I do to the stuff sloughed away during a facial or the strands on the floor after a haircut.

But if I do not fulfill my desire to have kids, and I never use my frozen eggs because some unforeseen circumstance prevents me from doing so—I decide I cannot go it alone and be a single mom but never meet the right person to be a parent with, some medical reason dictates I cannot bring a child to full term, I discover I cannot afford to thaw and fertilize the eggs, or whatever other reason may arise—I think it is safe to assume I will have very different feelings about those eggs. They will not be meaningless. They will not be just a few cells to which I have no attachment. They will represent what could have been but never was—an opportunity that slipped from my grasp. Unrealized hope and potential is, to me, always sad. But the unrealized hope and potential of my becoming a mom, when I was *this close*, when I did all I could to make it happen, all those injections and that invasive procedure and that tremendous financial and emotional expense—that would be devastating. In fact, I am getting teary-eyed even as I type this.

But I still have hope that the crazy, random events of life—all the unpredictable stuff that happens to us—will, in the end, break my way. You never know what is in store for you. That much is certain. So once you have hedged your bets and done all you can to ensure the future you want, why not choose to believe that only good things will come to you? Face the heartache of giving up on those eggs if and when that situation arises; do not suffer through it before you even know you will have to. That is my plan, anyway.

Next, we will start talking about *your* plans—but first, you will meet two more women who have been through this process (as I said, my voice certainly isn't the only one you should listen to!), and you will continue to see just how varied this experience can be.

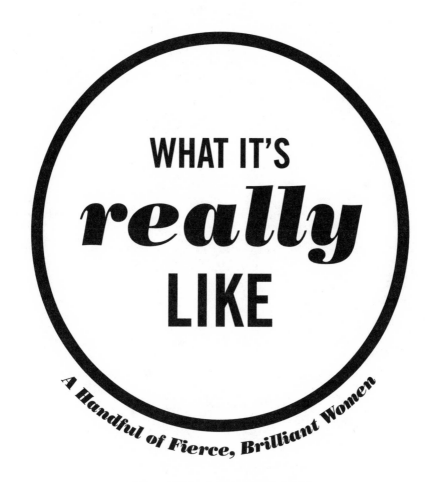

WHAT IT'S
really
LIKE

A Handful of Fierce, Brilliant Women

SHARE THEIR EXPERIENCES FROM
THE EGG-FREEZING PROCESS

You have already heard my experience of egg freezing, and bits and pieces of other women's experiences. And now, of course, I hope you are much more familiar with the process than you were before. But I think it is still worthwhile to hear exactly what the process stirs in the women who go through it, because I do not think you can make an informed decision without the down-and-dirty, no-holds-barred, nitty-gritty info. I also think you will benefit from hearing how their decision-making processes unfolded. After all, you might soon be in the midst of your own. And with that, I cede the stage to my fellow freezers.

AMELIA *had a pretty routine experience of the egg-freezing process—no complications, no real difficulties. But that ordinariness is exactly what makes her story so useful to prospective freezers. Even without any major hiccups, her experience was filled with conflicting feelings and logistical issues that needed her attention:*

"I don't really know how I heard about egg freezing—I assume in magazines, or online. I had asked my doctor about my options, and she was like, 'You're young, you're fine. Maybe at thirty-five.' She really just kind of dismissed me. It was like, 'Just live your life; don't put pressure on yourself.' So I didn't—but I also did *not* wait until thirty-five, as she had suggested. I think realistically I started pursuing egg freezing around thirty-three. First, I had that same doctor take my blood work, the AMH test. I started exploring options with a few fertility specialists in the Bay Area. I reached out to a specific one, and they sent me all the information about the procedure. I sat on it for like six months—all of it. I didn't even get the AMH test results. I wasn't ready yet, so I just sat on it. I think it boiled down to having enough money and time—I had neither. I thought, *How on earth can I afford to freeze my eggs?* I was living paycheck to paycheck at the time. I knew I needed to change jobs and make more money. And I did that. I was feeling fear about time running out, and I also felt that this was just practical. *If I can get the money and my body decides to cooperate,* I thought, *it's just a no-brainer.* I am a planner, and it felt like the responsible thing to do. Give myself a safety net. When I am ready to be a parent, I will have that as an option.

"The experience itself was good. I remember it being a very female-focused, female-centric time in my life; I realized one day that I wasn't talking to any men—just friends who knew what I was going through. That was kind of weird. Mostly the experience was just really all-consuming. My life revolved around my period, the injections, the bloating, the travel restrictions. And in my job I travel a lot. So actually before I went through all this, I told my boss, who is a man, about it. He was very caught off guard that I shared that with him, but I needed him to understand that I wasn't going to be able to travel. I mean, maybe I *could* have traveled—I probably could have, honestly—but I was going to the clinic sometimes three times a week for ultrasounds and blood work, and doing that is stressful enough, especially when you're going really early in the morning before work. To tack on business travel as well, plus the injections every night . . . that would have been a lot.

"It wasn't hard to administer the medication—but it *was* thousands of dollars of drugs, so I was very cautious. I remember I made an egg-freezing play list for when I gave myself the injections. Doing something every night at the same time was hard for me, because my life is very chaotic. My body did not respond to the medications as well as I had wanted it to. I would go into the clinic sometimes and they would bump up my medication, and then again the next visit. It kept going on like that, and it was just like, *When is this going to stop?* It was an overwhelming few weeks.

"But nothing unexpected really came up, except for the very last injection—the trigger shot. That surprised me. It was a *huge* needle I had to jab into my butt, and nobody brought that one up, nobody had told me how enormous that needle would be. But at that point I had given myself so many shots I was like, *Eh, what the hell.* I knew it was the end, so I just told myself it was like the grand finale at the end of the fireworks show. I went out with a bang.

"I'm very sentimental—movies, commercials, all that stuff makes me cry. I am a big crier. During that process I did cry a lot, but they were mostly good tears. But I did sometimes get pretty angry, just that I had to be in this situation. I would think, *I wish I did not have to do this. I wish I were already a mother. I wish I had a husband or a partner.* It was something I had to do, I felt, out of desperation, and it made me mad that I had to do it. God, I forgot all those feelings until right now. I am relieved it's over, and I am glad it was successful. To have this pressure taken off me is a huge relief. I was very lucky in that I generated quite a few eggs—that is part of why the doctors kept bumping up my doses, because I had so many in each ovary. But it was a result I was still less than thrilled with, because while they were able to take out nineteen eggs, unfortunately only thirteen were viable to freeze. So that was my one disappointment. I knew I had tons in there and was excited with how many and how big [they were], and . . . I was bummed to lose six that I had been growing. But thirteen eggs is good. It was a successful haul.

"If you have the money and your body will cooperate, and you want to have children but don't see them on the immediate horizon, then I would definitely recommend doing it."

LAUREN *had a slightly more anxious experience. However strange it may sound (and even she knew it was strange), she had a fear that harvesting eggs from her body might somehow reduce her fertility in* *the future. (It does not.) She also went through the process while in a relationship, and is currently in another serious relationship, which has added an extra layer of stuff to consider. Namely that her partner is not sure he agrees with egg freezing on a philosophical level:*

"I think I was around thirty when I started to consider freezing my eggs. Actually, my mom initially put the thought in my head. So even though I was angry that she brought it up, it was around then that a few of my friends wound up doing it. I thought about it for two years, because it was a big commitment, of course. And I finally did it when I was thirty-five.

"When I was weighing my decision, my biggest concern was irrational: *If I take out a bunch of eggs now, does that affect my potential fertility in the future? Does the procedure have an impact on your ability to naturally conceive? Will I be dependent on these frozen eggs?* That was a big fear of mine. It's definitely not medically true—it has no basis in fact. But we all have our own fears and concerns, and those were mine. I was a little scared about the process, too, because I didn't know what to expect. But it was pretty seamless. I think the biggest pro in the list of pros and cons was a sense of liberation. This is not an insurance policy, necessarily, because the eggs might not be good—there's no guarantee—but it did give me some peace of mind that while I wasn't in a position to have a baby today, at least there could potentially be some chance of it later.

"The experience was pretty seamless initially. For the first two days it was a little nerve-racking, just because I had never given myself shots but thankfully, my boyfriend was very involved in the process and pretty darn good with a needle. It was all fine right up until the egg extraction, because I ended up getting ovarian hyperstimulation syndrome. But in the end the procedure was pretty successful: I froze twenty-eight eggs out of a total of thirty-six that were harvested.

"I am increasingly convinced that I want to have children, and I want to do it before I turn forty-one. And I am in a committed relationship right now—we've been together for three years. I'm really hoping that we can get pregnant. He doesn't really believe in the science of fertility, which is interesting. That will be an interesting bridge when we have to cross it. Ideally, we won't have to; ideally, we can get pregnant the old-fashioned way, without having to use the eggs. He thinks there's something unnatural about getting pregnant with medical intervention, and that nature should be left to take its course. He has all these opinions because he doesn't really get that things don't always work out the way you think they will. So yeah, that will be interesting. Really looking forward to it—just kidding, I'm not at all. But yes, that's the hope, that I will be trying to get pregnant in the next one to two years, and that in the end I won't even need the eggs I froze."

VICTORIA *is among the few women in this book who found her happy ending, baby-wise: she has a very young son whom she conceived with donor sperm. But she too froze her eggs before she knew she would go forward with IVF (using fresh eggs), and her experience was just as unique as the others described here:*

"I really hadn't thought about my fertility until my thirties, when my friends started to have children and I hadn't met anyone yet. It dawned on me that they were in a very different position than I was. I began to realize I didn't have forever. I froze my eggs in my mid thirties. I haven't made use of the eggs yet, if I ever will. When I turned forty, I did IUI and IVF—two rounds of the former, one of the latter. They didn't work, so I did a further round of IUI with a new doctor, and that's how I had a little baby boy. He's seven months old now.

"I've lived in New York for eight and a half years—I moved here when I was thirty-four, and a year later, I froze my eggs. I think it's partially because living in New York sort of normalizes these things—it's something many people do here, whether or not they talk about it. And I am a very decisive person, so I knew instantly that it was the right thing for me. I couldn't see any argument for *not* doing it. I thought, *Well, the worst-case scenario is that I will spend the money and not need the eggs.* Which would just make it a very expensive insurance policy, and to me that's still valuable. Either way, it was definitely worth it to me.

"I wasn't afraid of the medical part of it. I didn't worry about the procedure, the medication aspect. In fact I quite enjoyed the administering of the drugs via syringe—I think I would have made a good drug addict. It was all very easy, except that during the egg harvesting I had an allergic reaction to the anesthesia. I woke up the next day and couldn't open my eyes; I had to have a strong dose of antihistamine and steroids, but then I was fine.

"Worse than that, though, was the experience I had with the first implantation, with my first doctor. I had done two rounds of IUI and one round of IVF with her, and I think she handled it all very badly. On the day they transferred the embryos to my uterus she walked into the room and said, 'It's a boy.' Well, first of all, I hadn't wanted to know the sex, so that was upsetting. And her saying that—a 'boy'—turned what had been a science experiment into a baby. It made me grow attached. And it made me think this was all a done deal, that all was well and I would be having a baby. So when the implantation was unsuccessful, it was so much harder to come back from. Of course, everyone I've told this to has been disgusted, saying I should sue. (I don't plan to.) In the end I went to a new doctor, this time at a big hospital, because I think that's what you need for this procedure: a big system, as opposed to a tiny, posh Upper East Side doctor's office, which is where I had started.

"I think they got about fifteen eggs. But in the end, when I was ready to get pregnant, my doctor advised me not to use them. They want you to hang on to those eggs until you really, really need to use them, and since I was still producing my own eggs, I didn't need to."

HEIDI, *whose opinions about egg freezing are incredibly insightful, froze her eggs several years ago but found that doing so changed her opinion about her own potential motherhood in a way she never expected. I will let her tell you:*

"I started considering freezing my eggs when I was about thirty-one or thirty-two. You hit thirty-one and you realize it's not happening. I started realizing that there was this underlying stress in my life, that I was putting pressure on myself because this *thing* hadn't happened, the thing being both the relationship and also the children that would come out of the relationship. The other thing that happened is that a couple I was really close to went through a horrific IVF experience, round after round after round. And they finally did have a kid. But it was still really hard. I was so close to them, and though I'd never say I experienced what they experienced, they didn't hide a lot from me. I saw a lot of what was going on, and it scared the hell out of me. And I was always afraid that I would reach forty or forty-two and suddenly my biological clock would kick in, because it hadn't kicked in at all by then, and I would really be pissed at younger Heidi for not getting it together. And this couple's experience was like this warning to me, because in their case I think the biological clock had just turned on all of a sudden for them, like *boom*. And I was just really scared of that.

"I wanted to take control, because I was also realizing that when I was dating I was putting a lot of pressure on that, thinking I had to get the dating thing right. That, and this fear of the future—those two things coming together made me finally decide when I was thirty-four to just do it, to freeze my eggs. That decision was a bit delayed. In the beginning I thought it was almost a shameful thing. I thought the reason I had to freeze my eggs was because I failed. I failed at relationships and I failed at getting my act together as a woman. And there was a year or so when I was rolling it around in my head that I didn't want to do it because of that sense of failure that I associated with it. And then something clicked in me where it went from being a failure decision to a control decision, an empowering decision. Like, *No, wait, actually I'm just going to do right by me.* And that's when I made the switch and decided to do it.

"Overall, during the process I had this feeling of gratitude, knowing that I'm in an economic position that I can do this, and never forgetting that. I think this healthcare system is so messed up, it's so much against women, and to think that you have to be privileged in order to have this sort of clarity and decision making in your life around your reproductive rights just feels very wrong to me. I went to Weill Cornell Medicine, so I was at a very good clinic. I was surrounded by some very wealthy people, and it was just this reminder all the time that I hope we're the trailblazers who can create a sense of normalcy around this so it eventually becomes something that can be adopted on a wider scale. I would love to give this type of freedom, this sense of calm I have, to other women.

"As far as the experience itself, the biggest thing I didn't anticipate is that when you're freezing your eggs you're making a proactive choice, but at these fertility clinics you're surrounded by women who are in a desperation moment. And the difference in energy and emotions was really shocking to me. You know, sitting in these rooms, because you have your morning checkup and you're going in almost every day at like five o'clock in the morning, and you're sitting in this room and these women are filing in and they are just desperate and strung out and stressed and hoping beyond hope. And I remember one time I was sitting in the waiting room and there were like 150 women waiting to do their morning check, and a woman comes in with a stroller, and you just felt this wave of yearning and sadness as soon as that kid started squawking. When women found out that you were doing egg freezing and not IVF, there was almost a sense of jealousy. I mean they were so supportive, and everyone was lovely, and I don't want to say it was bitchy. It wasn't bitchy. I just think you have to prepare yourself, because you're having the minority emotional experience and the women around you are having an incredibly heightened emotional experience; this is one of the most important things that has ever happened in their lives. And you represent to them the decision they didn't make or couldn't make because it wasn't available. It's going to feel a little weird sometimes. Sometimes I would shrink away from other women in the waiting room because I didn't want to talk to them. They would be like, 'Oh, I'm on my fifth round of IVF,' and I would be like, *Oh my God, you poor thing.* And that was something I didn't anticipate in the process.

"If we want this to become more widespread, obviously the cost needs to go down, or insurance companies need to better support it. So there's a systematic or societal change that needs to happen there. Although sometimes change comes out of the private sector, which can force government to make changes. But at the end of the day, it's about people respecting that women need this autonomy and this choice, and at what point in our society do we start to respect women like that? Part of that is women *demanding* respect. Part of it is people like us talking about it. I remember when I first started talking about freezing eggs people would start to whisper, and even my most powerful, awesome girlfriends felt dirty talking about it. And now I talk about it all the time, because I feel like just talking about it is really important.

"The second I got the phone call—I was at a Walmart in rural Pennsylvania with my boyfriend at the time, and I get the phone call from the hoity-toity Upper East Side clinic being like, 'You have fourteen eggs and they're really healthy; congratulations,' and this weight just fell off of me. It was almost physical. I think for the first time in my life I was allowed the freedom to really ask myself if I wanted to have kids or not. There wasn't this sense of gloom and doom."

HEATHER *was resistant to the idea of freezing her eggs—something I often hear from women who do not yet know much about the process, or who think getting pregnant will be easier than it is. But in the end, Heather decided to go forward with the procedure, after an encounter that woke her up to the reality of her situation:*

"I had always liked the idea of having kids, but I never met the right partner. The partner part was more important than the kid part. So for years I really didn't think about kids at all. Or if I did, I thought, *Well, celebrity so and so is having kids in her mid forties—I'm fine.* I only really started talking about it when a friend froze her eggs. At the time, I thought it was really extreme, mostly from a money perspective. Then I started talking about it with other friends, and was surprised to discover that others had done it. It's interesting, because you can know someone really well and then find out something like that; unless you're with her in the moment it might not be something you talk about.

"It all changed for me about two years ago. I started to think seriously about freezing my eggs. But my insurance, like that of most companies, doesn't pay for it, so it was all going to be coming out of my wallet. What's funny is that I had gotten my MBA a few years before, and paid nearly $150,000 in tuition without giving much thought to the cost, because the degree was so valuable to me. So I thought, *Why doesn't it bother me to spend that much on school, but [I'm uncomfortable paying] $16,000 for this?* There were decisions I was making about vacationing and school, where I was spending a lot of money that I wouldn't have even thought twice about. It was around then I realized I could do this. It was an insurance plan, in my mind—a just-in-case plan.

"I was turning thirty-nine around then. I had friends that had gone through a lot of fertility issues, and I knew that you often don't know how fertile you are until you start to try. So I went for a consultation—that was $600. Okay, so don't go out to dinner a few times and you're pretty much there, in New York. I thought, *I'll just go have her do an exam and see if I have eggs even to freeze.* The doctor came back with pretty self evident news: 'You have a thirty-eight-year-old uterus,' and she gave me an estimate that I would get eight eggs. They say that for every eight eggs, statistically, you get one child. So it was smart of the doctor to say that, because I ended up getting sixteen.

"The experience was fine. My friend who had also done it was there for the first injection. After stabbing myself with the syringe, she laughed and said, 'You don't have to do it so hard.' The anticipation of it was harder than actually doing it. I would say that you certainly get to a point where it's uncomfortable and you're just done with it. Almost every morning I was commuting to the far east side for my check-ins, which is hard to get to via subway, so it became just bit of an annoyance. I was traveling a ton for work around then, so taking two weeks out of my schedule to not travel felt like a big, hard commitment at the time. I also run, practice yoga and am mildly addicted to CrossFit, and so the not being able to work out thing was a big bummer. But now, looking back on it, I feel like it was the best way to spend two weeks: creating an insurance plan for myself.

"In the end, I'm so glad I did it, and I tell my younger friends that they should at the very least look into it. When they talk about fertility, I hear in them a lot of myself when I was their age. 'Oh, I'm only thirty-four, I'm going to wait a couple years.' But you should do it now! Your eggs are fresh. And you really never know how life will turn out. I look at myself today and I can't believe I'm forty and no closer to having kids.

"Then again, it's easy to say 'You should do this,' but I understand what you're like at twenty-five. At that age, you're not thinking that's where your money should go. So how do you ed-ucate that age group on why it's so important? I have a few very good friends in their early thirties, who I've said all this to a cou-ple times. But while I'm talking to them about a 'fertility insur-ance plan,' they don't even have a 401(k). It's tough when you have to make choices like that—they're trying to prioritize. So I talk to them, but I don't preach to them.

"The other day I was at a grad school alumni event, talking to a woman who's forty-five. She's dating people but not married. I'd asked her if she wanted children and she said she didn't know, and I offered up my information, told her I froze my eggs. She was like, 'Yeah, me too, fifteen years ago.' It was super beta then; she didn't get as many eggs as she probably would now. I felt like I was talking to a future self. She said, 'If you want kids, I would make that your number one priority, or you'll end up like me.' I thought, *So at what point do I stop hoping for this? At what point do you tell them to throw the eggs away?* My year has always been forty-five. So the fact that this woman was saying that at forty-five, going through that ques-tion of whether or not to keep them, that scared me."

ALISON *is deeply enamored of the idea of becoming a mother. In fact, it is often difficult for her to discuss the subject without tears. This process was, in many ways, an emotional one for her—which you will see when you read her powerful thoughts on the subject:*

"In your twenties you have the luxury of saying, 'I want to explore things; if this relationship doesn't work out, no big deal.' In your thirties it shifts. It becomes, 'I am dating to inevitably, hopefully, end up with this person.' You don't want to waste your time. For me, everything started to shift. *Where do I want to deepen my roots, where do I want to be? What kind of environment should I put myself in to meet someone?* Nowadays I'm even more conscious of who I'm dating. The desire to have kids has never been stronger for me.

"When I asked my doctor about fertility, she said, 'Here's someone we send people to. They do testing and analysis, baseline stuff. Why don't you call them?' So I called and set up an appointment (it took forever; they were incredibly booked up) and I had an honest discussion with the fertility doctor. 'Having my own children is a nonnegotiable for me,' I said. 'Be totally frank and honest with me. Looking at these numbers, what do you think?' And the doctor said, 'I think if you go back out there and try to find the right guy, and you walk back through my door a few years from now asking me to help you to get pregnant, there might not be much for me to work with.' I decided right then I was going to freeze my eggs.

"I knew nothing about the process. I think I've become so passionate about this because I did not hear anything about it at all, and I imagine all these women who would be helped by it but have no idea it even exists. I wound up undergoing the process twice, and my first round was brutal. From an emotional standpoint, and from a results standpoint. I thought I would go into this amazing, empowering experience and feel liberated, like, *I can go back into the dating world with this weight off my shoulders.* But it was such a disappointment—I had very few viable eggs. Again, going in, I had known nothing. I didn't know anyone who had gone through it, so I went in so blind, got wrapped up into the process, and it wasn't until halfway through that I realized my body was not responding. The doctor kept calling me, saying, 'We're not seeing much, but we'll keep going, and then have some appropriate conversations before retrieval.' They were basically like, 'If it doesn't make sense to do a retrieval, you can get some money back.'

"I think that was the first time I had this realization that here was something I thought I could control, and now I was sitting down looking at my body and being like, 'Why aren't you responding?' It was such a separation of mind and body. I was so angry and disappointed. I thought I would go through this and be so vocal,

I would tell all my friends; I wanted all my friends to rally around me. Looking back I was like, *I can't believe I told everybody.* My whole social circle would ask how it was going, and having to be honest with someone that it isn't going as well as you thought—I felt like a failure. I feel like there was a lot of vagueness at the center I chose, like I was a small fish in a huge pond. But there are other centers out there that are much more one-on-one, that do the emotional check-in.

"I did round two about a month after the first—but this time it was totally different. I got my head on straight, did a ton of research. The process is basically IVF, minus the fertilization with sperm and the embryo transfer, and while there's not a lot of conversation out there about egg freezing, there's *lots* of information out there for women doing IVF—stuff about how to increase your egg count, how to make sure your ovaries are in a good place. The role of acupuncture, supplements, things like that. If I had known all that the first time, I might have been better off—at least to have the knowledge, to have the choice to try these things leading up to the process. So I decided I would explore those things before round two. I would focus on my diet, I would exercise, I would get my body in tip-top shape. That was nothing like the time before, when I had been having martinis the day I started the process.

"Of course, I am not one to preach, and I don't want to give people false hope about what will impact their results. But I think my second-round results do say a lot. The first time I got two to three eggs. The second time I got fifteen. I will say that the doctor and I worked very closely together to figure out a very different protocol that second time. A lot of women don't have that option. Some women are like, 'I'm going in for one round, because that's all I can do.' But it isn't like going to your doctor when you have a cold. If you only go through the process once, it's hard for a doctor to know what your body will respond to. I think everyone was surprised that I responded so poorly the first time around. But I was really driven to have enough eggs to give me peace of mind, so I was like, 'If this doctor is saying to do another round, game on. If she is confident that this protocol will make a difference, I am going to believe her.' Given that this is one of my biggest desires in life, I knew I had to go for it.

"I'm a pretty results-driven, solution-focused person. I have been my whole life. The way I look at life and things I want is very much like, 'I want it, and here's the path to get there, and I am going to succeed.' And I had gone into the first round with that same attitude. Like, *I am going to win at this. I am young for this!* Even my OBGYN was saying, 'You're too young for this; you don't need to worry about this yet.' That boggles my mind now. Two other doctors I met with had said the same thing. I wish I could call them back and tell them they could not have been more wrong. I got two eggs. Two! And I was too young?

"So when I went back for round two, I made sure to be up front about what I had gone through, and I was like, 'Here are some areas of opportunity I feel you could be doing a better job at.' That first round really haunts me, still. Since then, I've had people ask me to talk them through it. I know one person in her mid thirties who went in, had this amazing experience, and got a ton of eggs. On the other side of the spectrum, I have a really good friend who's thirty-five, and she had a really similar experience to my first round. And she was so upset about it, she decided not to do it again. She is throwing in the towel. I realize this is everyone's individual experience. If that's not something she can go through again, I have to support that. I think when you start to look out there at what little is being written about this, all you really see are success stories. Of course it's easy to talk about success! But where are the rest of the people? Sometimes people get *no* eggs. There's a piece of the conversation that's missing right now. The truth of this process is not just 'Come on in and get that weight off your shoulders!' It's like, 'This is an option, and you need to know that there are different outcomes.'

"I think I was most surprised by how in tune and connected to my body I felt. Obviously the first round I was becoming connected to it in a negative way, which was hard and awful. But going through that helped me fuel the changes I made before the second round. I treated my body with such compassion that time. And you have to be very clued in, for almost two weeks, to what your body is doing. You have to give yourself shots, and that was hard for me—it's so weird to, like, make that stabbing motion into your own body. I remember thinking, *Oh my God, my head and hand are not syncing up. I need to shove this in my stomach, but I am so not used to the idea of doing this.* But what was so interesting was that over time it became such a moment with myself, those injections. Your entire kitchen counter is nothing but syringes and vials. It was shocking to me, but they have you mix the stuff up yourself, and you're like, *Wow, I'm a scientist now.* I think you get obsessed with the process. I was kind of sad it was over—it had become this moment when I was doing something for myself, and I got so used to that. It's a misconception that it's some big time-suck. I think women don't understand that this is really only like three weeks out of your life. You're not taking any time off from work—I worked all the way through the process, and then took one day off for the procedure.

"I'm lucky to have two parents who were like, 'We'll get you through as many rounds as you need to get enough eggs.' The day I found out the first round hadn't done that well, I remember my dad saying, 'We'll do four rounds if we need to.' It was so powerful that my father would agree that my ability to have children was that important. And of course it is always nice to hear a parent say 'We're with you every step of the way.' It isn't like that for everyone. I know several people who did it without telling their parents. In fact, many women I've spoken to said they don't often talk about doing it, because it was embarrassing, a personal choice, a taboo. I want to change that.

"I think there are a few things I've realized after this process. My desire to have children did not subside even though I froze my eggs. I thought it would become more back of mind, like, *Now I'm going to get back into dating and have fun.* That did not happen. I still feel the pressure and the need and the desire. I want to meet the right person, and I want to start that part of my life. My goal and my desire is to have children on my own and not necessarily to use the eggs. I would try on my own, and if I couldn't get pregnant, I would use them. My doctors would only make me go through about three months of trying naturally before letting me use the eggs. Honestly, I think it's just *healthier* for you to use this thirty-two-year-old egg.

"It has been a bit of an interesting exploration—dating after freezing your eggs, I mean. When do you tell someone about this, and when do you not? Originally I was so confident and proud of what I had done, and I was getting involved in the dating scene after moving back to San Francisco. I was telling these guys I was seeing all about it, and it wasn't long before I realized how many men did not understand it and actually were pretty turned off by it. I had a few different guys say, 'I think you should tone it down.' I was so surprised by that, because I was like, 'You should be stoked I did it! I'm not trying to have babies tomorrow—there's no pressure on you! If anything this should make me *more* attractive.' But what they hear is just like, 'You're talking about babies, babies, babies; you just need to stop.' So I've definitely struggled with dating in terms of when do I say it, and how do I say it in a way that doesn't scare someone away?"

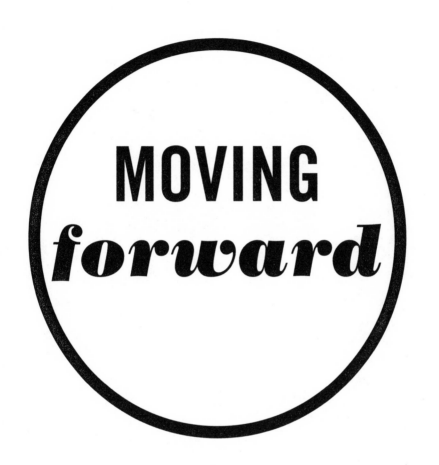

So now you know . . . a lot, actually! In fact, you probably know quite a few things you did not know before you picked up this book. You know that you did not learn everything you need to know about reproductive health in high school sex ed. (Actually, you did not learn *most* of what you need to know about that subject.) You know the major parts of your baby-making factory, and what each of those parts contributes to the process, be it hormone production or follicle growth. You know the nitty-gritty of egg freezing, right down to the daily details, and you have read several women's accounts of what they went through when they froze their own eggs, including my own. In fact, you probably know much, much more about me than you needed to—but hopefully my story has helped to illustrate my point.

Most important, you now know that you have options at your disposal to protect your fertility and to keep your options open. And whether or not you choose to exercise those options, at the very least, you are now armed with information that can change your future— and give you a great deal of peace of mind here in the present.

But here is the next step: learning how to exercise these options on a practical level. We have already covered the financial, logistical, and social issues inherent in egg freezing—now we are going to dig into those with a little more depth.

How do we go from the traditional notion of having babies the old-fashioned way to a brand-new paradigm—one in which more and more women are living independently for much longer, if not for the entirety of their lives? A paradigm in which, even when you find a traditional relationship, it often looks very different than it once did because both parties have equally important and meaningful careers?

There was a time when this was simply not the way it was. There was a time when one income was enough to support a family, and that income was almost universally the man's. Back in these good old days (and by "good old days," I mean the sad and oppressive days), people got married younger, and the man often worked while the woman stayed home and had babies, then raised them and looked after the house. Some couples still function this way, but it is no longer the sole scenario most young women aspire to or are offered. When women hold high and influential seats at the table, when the number of female CEOs is growing with every passing year, it is clear that our careers are equally important on both the micro and macro levels. (Admittedly, there is still an inexcusable pay gap between men and women doing the same work, which is unacceptable, and quite rightly the focus of many vocal and determined feminist activists. However much progress we have made, I would be remiss if I did not acknowledge this.)

Now, most women work for the same reasons, and with the same intensity, as their male counterparts. Granted, I live in New York City, which is not entirely representative of the rest of the country—many women in this country still stay home to raise a family while their husbands work—but even so, my reality represents the reality of a lot of other women too. I work because I need to earn a living, of course, but I also work because I love my job, and, yes, I love the money I make doing it. I work for my future. I work for the future of a possible family, but I also work for a potential future alone, where I age without the support of a husband or children.

I also work because I love the challenge of it. I work so I can travel, so I can go out for nice dinners, so I can feel accomplished, fulfilled, and independent. These are, I gather, many of the reasons men work. I am not just trying to get out of the house on weekdays. I am not just passing time until I find another partner. I am participating in the world, I am pushing myself as hard as I can, and I am getting paid well to do it.

This new paradigm is empowering for women, and I embrace

it wholeheartedly. And it has largely been driven and created *by* women. It has led to a generation of women who can do anything the boys can do . . . except, sadly, procreate deep into their golden years. And therein lies the issue. Because what this paradigm has also done is created a wide pool of women, that includes me, whose only option as it relates to having biological babies is to hold off, and then pay the price, both literally and figuratively, later.

So back to my original question: how do we, as a brand-new generation of women, make this equally brand-new paradigm, in which women are thinking about babies much later in life than they have in previous eras, work for us? How do we navigate this newly redefined culture such that we can become moms later in life if we so desire? I believe there are four relevant things to consider:

1. We need to acknowledge why we are delaying motherhood so we can better plan.

Earlier, I discussed the concept of economic infertility—the notion that babies are simply too cost-prohibitive for many women, even if they are gainfully employed—and how it often affects women in major metropolitan cities, where the cost of living (and child rearing) can be staggeringly high. Let's run down the statistics again: The percentage of first births among women aged thirty years or older increased from 5 percent in 1975 to 26 percent in 2010 (the most recent year for which these figures are available). Since 1970, the average age of first motherhood in the United States has increased from twenty-one to twenty-five, driven primarily by an increase in first children born to women thirty-five and older. It will not surprise you to learn that fertility challenges, which typically become more pronounced in women older than thirty-five, are more common as this average age of first births has increased.

And this trend, I am sorry to say, is not likely to change any time soon. Similarly, the cost of living continues to rise, particularly in those staggeringly expensive urban environments I mentioned, and the only way for us to keep up is to continue to pursue and work in high-powered, all consuming professions. Which essentially guarantees that this perfect storm of economic infertility and delayed pregnancy—too little money, and a challenging and demanding job that makes mothering difficult—will continue indefinitely.

So what is to be done? First up, you need to know this sooner than most women do, and certainly sooner than I did. If you are reading this at age twenty-five, for instance, take note—and start socking away the money now. If having a baby someday is important to you, make it as much a long-term financial priority as your eventual retirement, or the purchase of your first home. Do not—I repeat, *do not*—count on some future partner to be there to share half the cost of raising a child. Because there may come a time when you realize that partner is not coming, or that you no longer care so much about finding a partner at all, or that you never needed one in the first place—and if and when that day comes, you want to be prepared to foot the bill yourself, should you so desire.

2. We need to get over the idea that motherhood completes a woman.

As I conducted research while writing this book, I spoke to a wide range of amazing women. Some of these women never really had the urge to have children but were not entirely sure. Some of these women had known their entire lives they wanted to be mothers. Some of these women felt like they could take or leave this whole baby thing. Some were lesbian women, whose situation—and logistical reality, in terms of getting pregnant—is very different from mine. All these remarkable women were ambitious, smart, and successful, and yet very few of them had ever really spent time considering the upside of not having children.

And therein lies a problem. I had an interesting conversation about this with Rachel Abrams, founder of Turnstone Consulting and author of *Pins and Needles: What to Expect When You're Not Expecting*, a graphic essay about women navigating the world of fertility. She hit the nail on the head when she told me that the underlying panic women in their late thirties experience is largely driven not just by their biological clocks but by a lifelong lack of thinking about what life might look like without bouncy babies in it. Suddenly a huge turning point is staring them in the face—and they have to decide, on the fly and with little time left, what they really want. What is the script for the rest of her life if she does run out of time? And can that script be just as happy and fulfilling as the one that included babies?

Heidi said much the same thing but in another way. Before she froze her eggs, she says, "there was this biological gloom and doom I was carrying, this sense that I was going to mess something up, wait too long. That pressure, when it came off me, it was the first time I was able to ask myself with clarity if I actually wanted to have kids or not."

As far as we have come (I refer here to all that brand-new-paradigm, dawn-of-a-new-era stuff I mentioned a moment ago), there is still a very narrow expectation of what women will eventually do with their lives, be they CEOs or bank tellers, stay-at-home wives or movie stars, professors or janitors: they will, our culture unilaterally decides, have children. This is, in the eyes of many, nonnegotiable. The default setting. That is what we are supposed to want, and that is what we are supposed to do. Babies, in the eyes of society, complete a woman, and without children, women are seen as somehow not completely whole. Not just un-whole, straight up *sad*. This narrative of female worth and function is so insidious, you might not realize just how deep it runs in our collective unconscious. Especially because, as I mentioned, things *are* so different for women these days: so much progress has been made, and still, somehow, this absurd bias continues to dominate the way we think about women.

If you do not believe me, take a look at the nearest newsstand. Here you will find the perpetual lightning rod of childlessness shaming: that paragon of toned arms and enviable flat-ironed hair known as Jennifer Aniston. How many times has the media portrayed her as sad, lonely Jen, pining for a baby and missing her erstwhile, long-departed ex-husband? Or as Jen herself lamented not long ago in the *Huffington Post*, she is also frequently represented in the press as a baby-bump-sporting redemption story, even though she has never actually turned out to be pregnant. As though the second she *does* get pregnant, she will finally be whole, her life no longer a sad cautionary tale of thwarted dreams. Poor Jen, these publications declare. She lost Brad to that effortlessly fertile minx Angelina, who is apparently able to breed like some kind of Adderall-dosed rabbit (and who has adopted enough kids to fill out a soccer team). All the while, Jen has remained single (well, at least for a while; she is now married) and childless (at least at the time of this writing). Poor Jen, indeed.

Poor Jen? The woman is worth upward of $150 million. She is gorgeous. She gets to spend her days deciding which projects she works on and which ones she does not. She can travel the world. She has nobody to worry about but herself (and megababe Justin Theroux—whom I would happily worry about in Jen's stead, should she ever wish to take a break). She has slept with men most women only dream of being near, and she has deep and abiding friendships. She can do whatever she wants, whenever she wants. Why the hell would we think she is unhappy? Because she does not yet have a baby? I mean, what is all that marvelous, lucky stuff worth if you are childless? Ugh. Just in case it still needs to be said: *Women do not necessarily need to have a baby in order to be happy, complete, or worthy.*

Listen, I know this whole book is about fertility. And as you know by now, this journey started for me in the first place because I so badly wanted to be a mother (and am still in the process of trying to figure out if I truly do, at all costs, want a baby). But regardless of where I stand on this personally right this second, I think it is important to acknowledge that there can be an entirely different narrative for the millions of women who have run out of time or options—or the ones who never wanted the option to reproduce in the first place. Statistically and culturally speaking, having babies, or wanting to, is still the norm for most women. It is ordinary, in other words. So if that is *not* the path you take, you are therefore extraordinary. You are living an extraordinary life—and it is one that belongs entirely to you. There is real merit in that. Do not let anyone convince you otherwise.

3. We need to challenge our healthcare system to do better.

As far as women have come, some aspects of this culture remain, as I said, painfully behind the times. Few institutions in our society make this more evident than the healthcare industry. Insurance companies have, at best, simply failed to keep up with how many of us will start families later in life than we did in previous years; at worst, they have intentionally designed the system to make it impossible to get fertility treatments covered. Currently, only fifteen states have laws requiring insurance coverage for such treatments. A few other states have some laws requiring certain treatments around *infertility* (meaning they will treat the underlying issue causing infertility, but not actually cover the treatments required to get pregnant, etc.). And in exploring the possibility of being a single mom, I have discovered that our healthcare system fails single women (not to mention lesbian women and gay men) disproportionately.

I mentioned earlier that egg freezing is seen as an elective procedure and, therefore, is not covered by most health insurance policies. Can we take a moment to acknowledge something that really should not even need to be said? Reproducing—the human will to procreate, the need for a species to perpetuate itself—is not actually elective!

Leave it to Kate to sum this up eloquently—and forcefully. "The moral dimension of this is the most problematic to me," she says. "Declining fertility and fertility related to age are somehow a moral issue in the eyes of our culture. It's about virtue, women's virtue, in a way that a hip replacement or a failing heart or erectile dysfunction is not. They're all about aging, organs failing. Why is it different to say to women, 'Your ovaries are failing; that's okay, medicine has a solution for that', than it is to say, 'Your hips are failing; that's okay, medicine has a solution for that'? We don't say to people with heart problems in their fifties, 'Sorry, nature intended for your heart to fail.' We don't say to people who get cancer in their middle years, which is in many cases also an age issue, 'God intended you to have cancer; you're burdened nobly.' When I was struggling to get pregnant, someone said to me at work, 'Oh, maybe it just wasn't meant to be.' You just want to punch somebody."

In general, any sort of fertility treatments are rarely fully covered by insurance, and when they are, the provider often makes it nearly impossible to take advantage of these benefits if you are a single woman pursuing pregnancy on your own, with donor sperm. Why? Because with many policies, you have to prove that you are infertile by demonstrating that you have already attempted to get pregnant the old-fashioned way for a certain period of time before they will deign to cover a round of IVF. Which, of course, you *cannot* prove if you are not married or partnered. Say it with me now: "That is completely insane."

While we are still on the subject of deeply distorted cultural assumptions—like, for example, that all women (including rich, happy women named Jen) are supposed to want, and have, children—let's go ahead and tackle another one. What does it tell a woman that a health insurance provider will not cover a round of IUI for her if she cannot prove prior attempts to conceive—which is to say, by extension, that it will not cover her if she is not married or coupled? What can she read into the thinking behind that policy?

She can extrapolate that her desire to have a child is somehow less valid, less *worthy*, than that of her married or partnered counterpart.

And the fact that a woman for whom IVF is (ostensibly) covered can only pursue the procedure if she has already suffered a failure to conceive indicates that insurance carriers see reproductive intervention as some kind of final stop on the train, something to try only when all else has failed. A last resort, in other words. But what about the single women for whom intervention is the *only* resort, and not some last-ditch approach? What happens to them?

If this retrograde, thoughtless policy is not evidence of the damaging and denigrating messages women receive from our culture, I do not know what is. Maybe it is just me, but I really do not like being told, however indirectly, that my desire to have children is less valid because I am not married or partnered up. I would be willing to bet that other women do not like being told this either. Which means that this policy is something that desperately needs to change.

To say nothing of the fact that very few employers even offer this (limited) benefit in the first place. At the time of writing, there are only a handful of major companies—most notably, Apple and Facebook—that cover egg freezing (they also cover other forms of fertility treatment, and offer amazing parental leave policies), and companies who cover IVF or other forms of reproductive assistance to single women who do not have a formal diagnosis of infertility are also deeply in the minority. Only 25 percent of insurance policies cover fertility treatments of any kind (and you can be sure that each contains considerable fine print, nuances, and caveats). And while some progressive *employers* offer egg freezing as a benefit (part of your compensation package, if you will), almost zero percent of insurance companies cover the egg-freezing procedure for women intending to delay having children. Until this tide begins to turn—until a greater slice of American corporations wise up and face the reality that women are waiting longer and longer to have children, and will therefore need fertility treatments to make having a child possible—

many hopeful would-be moms will find that babies remain painfully out of reach for them. If that does not break your heart, and also piss you off, I do not know what would.

4. We need to recognize that it's a man's world—and then we need to start chipping away at that, stat.

I have wracked my brain, conducted seemingly endless rounds of research, and attempted in every other way I can to analyze why, in this progressive day and age, legislators and health insurance companies still make it nearly impossible for many women (and couples too—let's not forget that) to access reproductive assistance. There is a booming fertility industry out there that is continuing, year after year, to grow. And it is largely growing thanks to out-of-pocket costs that drain millions of dollars from American women and couples. People go into debt in hopes of conceiving a child, while the fertility and reproductive assistance industry just keeps extending its reach and bulking up its coffers.

According to the investment bank Harris Williams & Co., the total market for fertility services in the United States is between $3 and $4 billion per year. About $1.5 billion of that is accounted for by the pharmaceutical side of things, including the hormones and medications taken to stimulate ovulation. The remaining billions include the services that fertility clinics provide, such as tests, treatments, and follow-up care. Globally, the market is even bigger, worth between $30 and $40 billion worldwide. The largest markets for fertility services include Europe, Japan, Australia, and Brazil—in all likelihood because those markets provide more financial support to patients, resulting in higher demand.

The United States' fertility industry only accounts for about 10 percent of the global fertility market. Think about that for a moment. How can it be that a country with one of the largest per capita income levels on the planet, and some of the highest levels of consumerism, represents such a minuscule share of the fertility market?

It is simple, really. Whether out of ignorance or, one shudders to think, by cynical design, the cultural establishment in this country—those middle-aged (usually) men, conservatives, who are, and have always been, in power—are still the ones who make decisions about healthcare policies. They are still the ones whose legislative decisions steer how this country views social politics, and dictate what is and is not possible for millions of Americans. Sadly, the healthcare industry, the major insurance companies, and the legislative arm of our government are still run by an out-of-touch crew of people who only seem to agitate for change when said changes benefit *the problems they can relate to.*

In 2015, Planned Parenthood suffered a major public relations crisis, in which a disingenuous pro-life group fabricated a story about how several Planned Parenthood doctors were selling aborted baby parts for a tidy profit. (These claims were, in case you missed it, untrue.) Yet despite this sudden public uproar over the use of fetal tissue for scientific research, Congress had already explicitly approved its use to help develop treatments for diseases like Alzheimer's. So why the uproar? Because, at best, through the lens of the conservative establishment, Planned Parenthood is largely seen as a government-funded abortion factory, or at the very least, an organization that serves to provide birth control to sinful women who obviously should not be having sex. What they fail to understand is that Planned Parenthood provides millions of women (many of whom are living in underserved communities or cannot otherwise afford health care) essential reproductive health services.

Here is a little case in point for you. It took six years for the American government to finally make birth control nationally accessible for women in this country, what with all the pill's uncomfortable connotations of women having sex simply for enjoyment's sake. But on the flip side, how long do you think it took for Viagra to get approved by the United States Food and Drug Administration (FDA)—or to be covered by most health insurance companies? If you guessed "not very long at all," you would be correct: it took only two years. And do you think there was some public outcry about the purpose of that pill? You think some stodgy old senator was railing against this immoral misuse of medicine, whose sole purpose is to allow men who cannot get erections to continue having sex? I am guessing no! If a woman who cannot conceive wants to get pregnant, she better sock away a year's salary or more, because the medical establishment sure is not going to throw her a bone. But if a guy cannot get it up (never mind that at a certain age, is it really *medically necessary* for a guy to get it up?), he need only make an appointment with his general practitioner, and in short order, a prescription will be written, a small co-pay will be paid, and all will be right again in his undershorts. Because, for God's sake, we simply *cannot* let a man go without the pleasurable use of his penis—horror of horrors! At least not when the folks in charge are proud owners of penises themselves.

Which brings me back to my original point: It's a man's world. That cannot be denied, that is for sure. But I do believe that—with enough time and vocal outrage and unceasing agitation, and as many candid conversations about these subjects as we can stand to have— it *can* be changed. And it starts with each and every one of us.

It is up to us to talk openly about these issues. It is up to us to pass the word on to our fellow ladies, and get them talking too. It is up to us to ask our companies and legislators to make this form of healthcare coverage—this life-changing opportunity—as available to us as it ought to be. And it is up to us to take control of our reproductive futures, to ensure that we preserve as much of our agency and options as we possibly can. Do that, and you lead by example. Do that, and you drive demand. You have more power than you think you do. So use it, girl. Be a vocal consumer, an educated citizen, and refuse to back down until you get your way. You do this every day at work and at home—that is just part of being a strong woman. Now is the time to start doing it on a more public scale, for your own good and for the good of your fellow ~~man~~ woman.

The way you spend your life, and the existence of the life you want to bring into this world, depends on it.

Which is why, on the following pages, I am going to provide you with exactly the script you need to follow to start taking charge of your own fertility—whether you are visiting the gynecologist for your annual checkup, walking for the first time into an egg-freezing consultation, or simply going forth into the world to keep on living your life. In other words, we have, at this point, covered pretty much everything you need to know. So now let's talk about what you can, and should, do with that very important, empowering information.

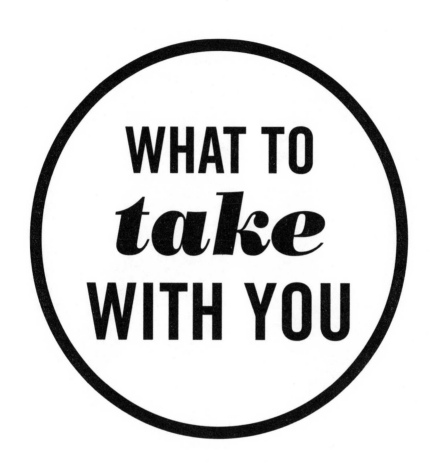

WHAT TO *take* WITH YOU

1. To the gynecologist's office

There are certain annual traditions in which we all take part. The year's first glass of champagne, just after midnight on New Year's Eve. The year's first glass of summer rosé, sometime after Memorial Day (or whenever the first warm day allows you to sit outside at your favorite bar or restaurant!). And, at some point between January and December, we all make sure to head to the gynecologist's office for what we call our "annual." (Or at least I hope you go each year, for the sake of your lady parts' health and well-being! Okay, lecture over.) And when we do make that visit, we are hopefully asked a few questions about any plans we might have for our ovaries in the coming year. The dialogue usually goes something like this: "Are you sexually active?" your doctor asks. "If so, are you monogamous? If not, how many sexual partners do you have currently? Do you use protection?" Which leads right into the big one—and, for our purposes, the most relevant one: "Do you plan on trying to get pregnant any time soon?"

Here is where things get a little tricky. Say you are in your early twenties. Your answer to that question is likely going to be something between a scoff and a grimace—hell no, you are not trying to get pregnant! (At this point, you are mostly just trying to make it to your next paycheck without eating goldfish crackers for dinner.) Say you are in your mid twenties. By now, you might not roll your eyes *quite* so far back in your head upon being asked this question, but you may still give the doctor a resounding "No." (You are probably eating actual meals by now, too—but you still may not be in any hurry to procreate.) Finally, say you are in your late twenties or early thirties. Now your answer to this important question may shift: depending on where you are in your professional and romantic life, you might say yes or you might say no. If you say yes, you will probably be whisked off into a whole other conversational realm, where such topics as timed intercourse, ovulation kids, genetic testing, AMH levels, and family health histories are likely to be covered. Congrats! You are well on your way to an informed, well-guided reproductive future. And for our purposes, you are pretty much off the hook for the moment—so go ahead and feel free to skip past this section.

But if you again answer that, no, you are not planning to get pregnant in the coming year, I am afraid you have a little more work to do. Your conversation with the gynecologist needs to continue. You can no longer let your resounding "No" be where the chat comes to an end.

First off, you will need to make sure to highlight your age. "I am ___ years old," you might start by saying. "Should I be considering the health of my ovaries and eggs?" This is the part where, if you are especially young—younger than thirty, say—your doctor is likely to throw a scoff right back to you, and then say something like, "No, no, you still have plenty of time." As you have learned, this is a common refrain among gynecologists. Warning: Do not accept this as an answer! Why? Because as we have discussed, it may very well do you, and your future fertility options, a tremendous disservice. The question itself—should I be considering this?—is actually something of a sneaky misdirect, because of course you should. Assuming you are already an adult, there is no such thing as "too early" when it comes to your fertility; the earlier the better. So if your doctor threatens to blow you off, here is what you come back with: "I want to be proactive about my fertility," you might say. "I would like to know sooner rather than later if my ovarian reserve or fertility potential is in any way compromised, so I can make an informed decision about how to proceed."

Just so you are fully prepared, the forcefulness of these statements may very well raise an eyebrow or two—most gynecologists are not used to hearing young women speak with such an informed tone about their own fertility. (In fact, most of them are not, as a rule, used to talking to a patient about fertility at all, until said patient's pregnancy is imminent, already existent, or frustratingly *nonexistent*.) But now you know that you need to be persistent. In fact, take it from Kate, who let her own gynecologist shut down the conversation when Kate was in her mid thirties.

"My OBGYN, who's a woman, was distinctly uncomfortable having this conversation with me," she says. "When I asked to have my levels tested, she receded, even to the point of pushing her chair back, and said, 'You're thirty-five, thirty-six; you should just go for it. I don't want to tell you that you should get panicked about this. You're perfectly healthy, I've been seeing you for years; let's not panic ourselves.' That was the context when I asked her to run fertility tests on me. I wanted to know my numbers, and she persuaded me not to do the tests. I think she felt very exposed—she wasn't trained for this. I don't fault her for it, because she was a warm and caring and knowledgeable doctor; she just didn't know how to have that conversation, and didn't know the right thing to do and felt like she was on ethically slippery ground. So as a result of that, I let myself be persuaded, and that was why I didn't pursue egg freezing."

This is exactly why we need to show our doctors that we are serious about this subject, and do not plan to shut up until we have the information we want.

And what information is that, exactly? What you are after, at this stage, is a preliminary read on your all-important FSH and AMH levels. So what you might say is, "May I please have my FSH and AMH levels tested so we can have an informed conversation about my ovarian reserve?" Now you will have dropped the hammer. Because once you show that you know exactly what information you are after, your gynecologist is likely to take you more seriously, and go about getting it for you.

Many doctors will be able to conduct these tests right there in the office or clinic; others may require you to visit another physician or a lab for these tests to be conducted. If it is the former, great! That is super easy. Many gynecologists take your blood to test for STDs on occasion—so when they do, just ask them to run the additional test. If insurance does not cover it, pay for it (then raise hell!).

After a short period of time—maybe a week or so—you will receive the results of your AMH and FSH tests. If your doctor tries to merely send you these results and let you make of them what you will, or says, "I'll just call you if something turns out to be wrong, but if everything is fine you won't hear from me," do not let him or her off that easy. Go back to the office or clinic and have a frank discussion with him or her about what these results mean. "Are you surprised at all by these results? Are they typical of, or unusual for, women my age?" If he or she says, "No, these look just about right," that is great news—congratulations, you now know that your reproductive future is looking relatively rosy. Now, of course, it is on you to continue having those numbers tested as time passes—again, do not let your doctor off the hook. You need to continue being your own advocate, because it is unlikely that your doctor is going to simply ask if you want to test these levels again a year or two down the line.

Conversely, you may decide—and it would be an entirely rational decision, as we have discussed—that however fabulous your levels are right now, you would still like to preserve your eggs in case things happen (because, you know, they often do). If that is the case, go you: you should win a medal for cool-headed pragmatism.

Now we come to the somewhat harder scenario. If it should become clear that your numbers are in some way dismaying or surprising to your doctor, you once again have a little more work to do.

First, you might ask for a more nuanced interpretation of your results. "Can you please explain to me exactly what these numbers mean?" Your doctor, if he or she is *worth* being your doctor, should walk you through a few things: the numbers he or she was hoping to see, the numbers he or she is actually seeing, and the significance of the gap between the two.

We have just reached the thorniest part of this hypothetical conversation. Do not feel like you need to make any decisions about next steps right there in the moment. Do not be *pressured* to make any decisions right there in the moment. Go home and mull over what you have just learned. Talk to your friends, your parents, and/or your partner, if you have one (and particularly if this partner is invested in your ability to have children). Figure out what is really important to you. You may discover, after all this mulling, that you do not feel a pressing need to have children, after all. You may discover that you feel the best way to proceed is to let nature take its course, and, as such, you do not wish to take steps to preserve your fertility, instead allowing the fates to decide if and when you will ever have children. (That, too, is perfectly okay.)

But maybe, after some thought—or maybe in the moment, depending on your levels of decisiveness and certainty—you will decide that having a child is incredibly important to you, and will decide right then and there to initiate the next phase of the conversation.

First, open with a simple question: "Knowing what we now know, is there anything I can do to increase my odds of getting pregnant in the future?" There are a variety of answers your doctor may give you. He or she may advise various changes to your lifestyle—exercise more often, drink more water, stop drinking alcohol or smoking cigarettes or consuming trans fats or mainlining caffeine. He or she may also advise a few key shifts in your diet. (Dozens of foods—everything from sesame seeds to salmon—are believed to increase egg health; you can find extensive lists of these foods online, if your doctor does not happen to mention them.) He or she may recommend acupuncture, fertility massage, self-massage, stress reduction, or a nutritional supplement to increase your ovarian reserve and overall odds of getting pregnant.

But let us not forget that you are also someone who has just read this book. You are armed with knowledge. And so once your doctor has finished telling you about the ability of halibut or turmeric or broccoli to increase your egg health, you may find yourself asking something like this: "Should I consider a medical means of preserving my fertility?"

There are some physicians who will view fertility preservation as the nuclear option. In other words, those eyebrows might start to rise once again. Your doctor may advise you to try less invasive and involved strategies—changing your diet, increasing your level of exercise, and undergoing acupuncture are all thought to influence fertility—before seriously considering something like freezing your eggs. He or she might advise you to put off thinking about egg freezing until every other method has been exhausted. But here is the important thing to remember: Yes, your doctor is a doctor. You, in all likelihood, are not. (If you do happen to be a doctor, well done! You probably do not need my help at all.) But the fact remains that you are also the one and only inhabitant of your body and your life, which means that your doctor—even with all his or her expertise—does not get to make the final decision about how you proceed.

So if what you really want to do is freeze your eggs—if you think your numbers merit that, or if it simply feels like the right thing for you in terms of your peace of mind—but your doctor attempts to dissuade you from considering it, make it clear that you will not be discouraged. Ask for his or her help. This "help" can mean different things. It might include referring you to a trusted fertility specialist or to a reputable egg-freezing clinic in the doctor's rolodex. Or it might mean working with you to develop a more multi-pronged approach: Maybe you will indeed decide to make some lifestyle changes—and *also* freeze your eggs. Maybe you will set up future AMH and FSH tests to monitor the progress your ovaries are making as you tweak your diet and habits and decide what, if anything, to do next based on those results.

2. To an egg-freezing consultation

If you have read this far, you are likely thinking seriously about freezing your eggs. Kudos—you are in excellent company. (Though, of course, I am biased.) When you visit the egg-freezing clinic or fertility specialist's office, you will need a similar script to follow, if only to make sure you do not forget to ask anything important or mention what really matters to you, and what your goals are.

And if you are here, you have already mastered one of the hardest parts of this process: taking proactive control of your fertility future. So now you find yourself in the next phase of the process. First of all, you will need to start by finding the right fertility center. (For starters, you can check an individual center's success rates by visiting sart.org, the site for the Society for Assisted Reproductive Technology.) Then make sure you feel comfortable with the doctor you find, on a personal level. I loved mine right away, which was important to me. You want someone who will be honest and straightforward, who will not patronize or condescend to you, and who you generally like talking to. Read up on their success rates, of course—but trust your gut about them too.

Landing in this part of the fertility universe may well be intimidating, even after you have learned the many ins and outs of the procedure. It might also be tremendously emotionally difficult. You met several women in this book who said how angry, sad, and disappointed they were to reach this point. You may be feeling very much the same way. After all, this may not be the outcome you expected or hoped for. (However, if you are doing this proactively, before ever trying to get pregnant at all, you may experience none of these emotions, or you may be feeling apprehensive or anxious, or you may be feeling something else entirely. In any case, congratulations on making a wise decision.)

Either way, what you are about to consider is a big decision, and it can represent a major turning point in your life. It certainly determines a whole lot about your future. Believe me, I get all that. But keep in mind that while all this science and medicine is totally foreign to us normal humans, this is what fertility clinics *do*. If you have picked a good one, with reputable doctors, this will all be relatively easy for them. Remember, it is just a manipulation of your menstrual cycle. There will be some hormones to ensure you lay a lot of eggs, and some blood tests and ultrasounds along the way to make sure you are on the right track, then a simple surgery at the end. Easy, right?

Yes, but go in prepared. Your initial consultation will probably begin with the doctor taking your medical history, which will involve him or her asking questions about previous pregnancies, miscarriages, attempts to get pregnant, failures to get pregnant, any family history of infertility, medical problems, surgical history, medications you are on, allergies, and a whole host of other questions; reviewing the AMH and FSH test results sent over by you or your gynecologist (and probably testing you again, as these results can change depending on how much time has elapsed since you first had those tests done); and asking about your goals and objectives, in terms of your future fertility, your wish to have a child (or children), and when you might go about this. This will likely also involve asking personal questions about your relationship status, sexuality, and sexual practices. So be ready to give those answers, even if they make you uncomfortable. They are important.

There are a few reasons why this initial conversation is so crucial. Your doctor is trying to explore and understand the greater context of your desire to potentially freeze your eggs. Are you considering this procedure because you want desperately to become a mom, and worry that you will not be able to do so naturally? Are you doing this because you do not fully know yet if you want to be a mom but merely want to preserve the option? Are you with a partner who may, you think, wind up being the coparent of your potential child? Are you single but hope to find such a partner? Are you single but have zero interest in (or hope about) finding such a partner? These questions matter, because they influence later decisions you will need to make during the process.

You should also be ready with what exactly you want, and why you want it. Here are a few sample statements:

"I am certain I want to have a child or children someday, and I hope eventually to meet a partner to coparent with."

"I am certain I want to have a child or children someday, and I am not interested in, or counting on, parenting with a partner."

"I am not entirely certain I want to have children someday, but I wonder if that might change if I should eventually meet a partner to coparent with."

"While my AMH and FSH levels are reasonably good, I believe in hoping for the best but planning for the worst, and I would like to have this option available to me in the future, should I ever need it."

And so on, right through all the various combinations and permutations and many, many variables that may influence your decision.

Bear in mind that you are, obviously, far less likely to encounter the same brand of surprise or dismissal from an egg-freezing specialist that you might have at your gynecologist's office. After all, these doctors are more than happy to help you get the ball rolling on this procedure—it is what they do, after all, and they believe wholeheartedly in its efficacy and value. But that certainly does not mean you can simply kick back and let them make all the relevant decisions for you. While a certain amount of deference to your doctors is a good thing—they are, after all, doctors, who probably know a whole lot more about these subjects than you do—you do have to make sure that you are participating fully in the process, making clear your desires and hopes and circumstances throughout. It is important to ask the doctor how many egg freezing and thawing procedures they have done with women's own eggs (not donor eggs). Although many clinics around the US have done a good number of freezing procedures, only a small portion have a good number of live births from the procedure to report. Ask specifically how many babies have been born as a result of women thawing their own eggs. Because this is a fairly new procedure, if the number of live births is less than 35, you might consider shopping around for clinics with more experience.

And if it is important to you to have plenty of hand-holding and encouragement—an emotional cheerleader, in other words, to guide you through what can be an emotional and taxing process—that is something you need to make clear. Because the truth is, not every doctor or fertility center is equipped to provide that. Doctors are people too, and because some people are more nurturing and supportive than others, these traits also tend to vary among physicians. So be up front with your expectations about your doctor or fertility center's involvement throughout the procedure. You might ask questions similar to these:

"If I have any questions or concerns throughout the process, will I be able to reach you, or someone else at the fertility center, whenever I might need to?" (The answer should be yes. My center, for instance, offered twenty-four-hour care; make sure yours does as well.)

"How involved will you be in the proceedings? Will I be working mostly with you, or with a team of nurses or other colleagues of yours?"

In many cases, you will not always see the lead doctor at the practice, or your primary fertility doctor at every visit—and that is as long as he or she is still the one reviewing your blood work every day and giving recommendations and suggestions on protocol. And as long as you can talk to him or her if you need or want to.

Now that you have a better sense of your doctor's commitment and involvement, which is crucial—and bear in mind that this is not a one-size-fits-all proposition. (For example, Victoria says she much preferred the large, factory-like atmosphere of a major hospital to the small, hoity-toity fertility clinic she had initially visited. To each her own!)

There are still a few more things to discuss. First up, whether or not you wish to freeze your eggs as eggs, or as fertilized embryos. Your doctor might not ask this if you are single—he or she may assume you will want to freeze your eggs as eggs, because this is the more typical procedure. So if you have questions about what the better option is for you,

you should nudge the discussion. As we discussed earlier, this decision depends largely on how you envision your future—namely, whether or not you hope or intend to use your frozen eggs alone or with a partner.

Once it is clear that you will be going forward with the procedure, you will need to consider several logistical issues: Will you be able to make it into the office every other day for blood work? Will you be able to take a couple days off from work for your retrieval procedure? How comfortable are you with needles, as you will need to self-administer these drugs multiple times a day? And some questions the clinic will definitely ask you: How do you intend to pay for this? Do you need advice about financing? And then there are the ancillary, but still necessary, subjects still to cover: where your frozen eggs will be stored, who will drive you home after your retrieval, and a dozen other little things. The good news is that this will hopefully all feel at least a little familiar to you because you have read my story, and the stories of other women, in this book. That firm base of knowledge will give you a leg up at this consultation, and throughout the procedure.

But there are some topics of discussion that may be more difficult for you to grapple with. Chief among them is the question of what the fertility center or doctor should do with any oocytes you do not wind up using; at some point in the process, you will be asked this. Do you want to donate them to be used in scientific research? Do you want to make them available to a couple or a woman who might be able to use them to create a baby? Do you simply wish for them to be discarded? It may seem premature to have this discussion—You may not intend to use these eggs for a long time, so how can you possibly know how you will feel about this years from now?—but you should be ready to have it just the same.

I want to address the women who may find—as did one woman discussed in this book—that her ovarian reserve is already so depleted, and her ability to create more eggs so limited, that egg freezing is not an option. You may be facing down a doctor who is saying he or she simply cannot help you. Perhaps this is because your age makes you an undesirable candidate. Perhaps it is because, for whatever reason, your ovaries are lying down on the job and the doctor feels they are unlikely, even with medical intervention, to produce a substantial number of viable eggs. I know I have just spent pages upon pages telling you to demand satisfaction from doctors who may try to shut you down—but there is an unfortunate reality to face here, and it is the sad truth that not every woman who desires a child is in a good position to freeze her eggs.

If your doctor tells you that you are among these women, by all means, get a second opinion. But—once again—do not let your desire to be told what you want to hear drive you to denial or, worse, into a costly and potentially fruitless procedure. What have I been saying, again and again, throughout this book? Options are everything. You are at your strongest when you have agency, and when you make the conscious choice to exercise it. And as devastating as it might be to hear that you may never bear your own children, you do have options. You can adopt, foster, use a surrogate, or make use of donor eggs. You can make your dream of being a parent real, if that is truly what you want. The way it finally happens may not look the way you always imagined it would. But it can still be wonderful. So please do not let anyone take away your hope—however grim things may look to you right now, this does not have to be the end of the story.

For those of you who find that this procedure *is* the right way to go, your story, too, is in some ways just beginning. Once you and your doctor have sorted through these endless questions and many thorny topics of discussion and you have decided to proceed, you will officially begin your egg-freezing adventure. You have my undying admiration and respect. You are doing something difficult but worthwhile. You are doing something that is potentially complicated emotionally, and yet so simple in its profound logic: this procedure will allow you to freeze your eggs in time, bringing you more options than you would have had prior. That is a remarkable, thrilling, magnificent thing. And so I say, once more, congratulations to you for making a wise and proactive choice.

3. From this book—and my twisty turny journey

If nothing else, I hope you take from this book—and me, a woman who has explored every aspect of this topic (and still is not sure how her story ends!), the following advice:

You should do whatever it is you want to do, whenever you decide to do it. No, I mean it. This is the crux of the matter. This is what it all comes down to when all is said and done. (And because we are at the end of this book, almost all *has* been said and done.) The belief that you should have the freedom to do as you like with your fertility is exactly what made me write this book—it is why I want you to have these pages of information and perspective at your disposal, why I want you to hear these stories of women who have been there before you, why I want to hit you with sobering statistics and rage-provoking facts about this country's healthcare system—so you can, come what may, be prepared enough to do what you want when it comes to your journey through your reproductive years, whether that leads you to the pursuit of baby making or to somewhere else entirely.

Of course, this will not always be easy. In fact, if I have made anything clear in this book, it is that these issues will *rarely* be easy to navigate.

Take me, for example. You know my story. You know I probably want to have a child or children. You also know that I do not know exactly how, or when, or even *if*, that will happen. I find myself, as so many women do, at a major crossroads.

Because while I can afford to provide a nice home for a potential child (or two), what I simply cannot afford is round after round of fertility treatments. (Unless lots of people buy this book! So please buy many, many copies. Think of it as your contribution to my potential future child.) This is true for so many other women—it might well be true for you. And that poses a huge societal problem. There are hordes of women out there who want to have babies. Women who would make amazing moms. Women who have had to work just as hard, just as much, and for just as long as their male counterparts, and who therefore did not get the chance to have kids during their prime baby-making years. Now, as a result, they cannot have those kids without some reproductive assistance. Yet these are women who also cannot afford to go through one or three or five rounds of treatments, and whose insurance either does not cover fertility treatments or, just as inexcusable, forces these women to jump through hoops to make use of the benefits to which they pay into. That is, by any definition, a broken system. Why do we allow it to continue?

The fact of the matter is a medical procedure that helps perpetuate the human race by allowing us to procreate in this new era of older parenting should not be likened to a boob job—which is essentially what is implied when the healthcare industry deems egg freezing and other fertility treatments as "elective."

When I froze my eggs, every piece of paperwork I had to fill out, every last insurance-related question I had to answer, reminded me that this procedure was indeed "elective." I suppose, in the minds of the people writing up those forms and asking those questions, my only other option would be to simply let my ovaries wither and die without ever being given the opportunity to produce life. And why? Just because I did not happen to meet the right guy in the time frame *they* deemed appropriate? How does that make sense? It does not.

This "elective" categorization would seem to assume that procreation is something we women simply decide we want to do for fun. But if you are someone who wants very much someday to have a baby, you already know that this desire goes a whole lot deeper than that. While many people choose not to be parents, choosing not to be a parent does not mean that for many others procreation is not a primal, natural, undeniable instinct. Wanting children is not a silly thing. This is not some frivolous undertaking. We are not hoping to give birth so we can have a little doll to dress up, or a tiny friend who looks just like us (though I would not mind a mini-me). This is important work we are trying to do! Maybe the *most* important work, continuing-of-the-species-wise. Having babies is how the human race persists. That is no small thing.

While having babies is important work, reality often intrudes. As a result, many of us have to put parenthood off for a while— sometimes a long while—because we get so busy making a living and becoming successful, productive, contributing members of society. This is not through any fault of our own. Waiting does not make you a failure. But it does sometimes mean we may need a little help getting pregnant once we *are* ready to take on parenthood. And that need is in no way the same thing as, say, waking up one day and deciding we want bigger boobs or fewer crow's-feet. *That* is the definition of "elective" in my book—undergoing a breast augmentation or having some kindly doctor inject your face with Botox so you can look a little bit younger. (Please do not misunderstand, Botox is my friend—I am not judging.) I believe that those far more unnecessary procedures cannot in good conscience be lumped in with one's ardent desire to bring a life into the world. Call me crazy, but I just fail to see how they are the same. (Of course, I do not begrudge you your desire, if you have it, to get your boobs lifted or brows decreased— just saying it is not *quite* on par with the desire to have a kid or two. You understand.)

I wrote this book at an interesting, and somewhat confusing, point in women's history. We have never been in a better position, in terms of the options we have at our disposal and our drive and ability to make use of them. We can go for what we want. We *do* go for what we want. And, best of all, we often get it. Compare that to the circumscribed way in which your mother or your grandmother or her mother had to live—think of the choices you get to make every day that those women simply never had the chance even to consider. In that sense, we have come a tremendously long way, and that cannot be glossed over or ignored.

But all that remarkable progress can distract, I think, from how much progress still has to be made. We have so much left to ask for—no, make that *to demand*. Equal wages, access to abortion services, the ability to go ten minutes without seeing a woman objectified or belittled or denigrated on-screen or in print. We cannot let ourselves believe that we live in a fully evolved society, in which all the great strides we have made as women mean there is not still more work to do.

Okay, I know how I sound. Right about now you might be thinking, *Jesus, lady, we are just talking about freezing your eggs, for God's sake. Who do you think you are, Gloria Steinem?* Well, no. And I do not mean to paint myself as some feminist hero. (Though I *am* a feminist, and, unlike some other, more cautious people, I am certainly not afraid to use that word—and neither should you be.)

However, I do think of egg freezing, and the way our society views reproductive assistance in general, as a microcosm of the way women are looked upon in this often deeply damaged culture of ours. And I also believe that changing one thing can eventually help to change everything. Reproductive control is the ultimate form of feminism. So—follow my logic, here—if we can normalize egg freezing, and if we can make that a valid option for more women, we can normalize the conversation around delayed baby making and fertility assistance in general. And if we bring those topics more firmly into the cultural conversation, we can also start talking about why it should be that women often have so little support when it comes to child having and child rearing, both at home and at work. We can shift something relatively small, and then that shift can beget other shifts, and when all these seemingly small shifts reach a critical mass, their combined impact will force our society to look at the greater problem, which is that public policies, societal expectations, and the stories we are told over and over are not keeping up with—and do not reflect—how women actually live today.

Feminism is and always has been about choices—the extent to which we have them, and how much freedom we have to exercise them. Your fertility is, of course, a part of your life that is extremely private, and yet the way we choose to make use of it has the power to drive public change. No, I am not Gloria Steinem, but as you might recall, she and women like her popularized the phrase "The personal is political," and that adage is as true of your fertility as it is of your decision to work outside the home or demand the same pay as your male colleagues. What you do in your life sends a message to the world. And because reproductive rights remain a hot-button issue in this country, what you do with your uterus and ovaries matters more than you might think. However you choose to navigate your reproductive life, never forget that.

But okay, fine—let's set all that heady politics and feminism and cultural change stuff to the side for the moment, because while it *is* undeniably important, it is not the *only* aspect of this discussion that is important. As I said, what it all comes down to in the end is what truly matters to you. Not your mother, not your friends, not your husband or partner—but *you*. If you want to have a baby—or babies—I want you to be able to. I want you to know more than I did, and more than many of my friends did. I want you to know more than your gynecologist tells you in a fifteen-minute visit, and I want you to know it in time for the knowledge to make a difference. I wrote this book because I felt cheated by my own lifelong ignorance, by how little I knew about the process and business and hard, cold biological reality of baby making. And I do not want that to be true for you.

For a variety of reasons this culture has, in all likelihood, denied you the information you need to make informed, proactive decisions about your reproductive future. If you have reached your mid to late thirties ill-informed, you have been cheated. Your sex ed teacher (who may have been, as is often the bizarre custom, your gym teacher—because obviously someone who oversees a kickball game is qualified to educate you about your ovaries and their contents) almost certainly left out the many nuanced things you need to know in order to plot the course of your reproductive future. In fact, you have been taught all kinds of faulty things. You were probably taught, especially in high school, to be careful, because you *will* get pregnant if you have sex. Your doctor's eagerness to put you on birth control combined with the images we see every day in the media of older, celebrity moms probably taught you that it is easy to get pregnant at just about any age. The stories you were told by Hollywood and Madison Avenue taught you that you must adhere to one narrative of motherhood—meet great guy, have kids, fulfill ultimate womanly destiny—which may or may not fit the reality of your life or what you wish for it. Your health insurance company taught you that you deserve, and will likely get, zero help in doing something so organic, so natural, so essential to human life. The silence of other women in your position taught you that discussing egg freezing and IVF and the deep, punishing sadness of infertility in general is somehow shameful or verboten—that these are experiences you must suffer through quietly, and often alone.

I hope we can start to unlearn all that. If this book can dispel even just one of those one-sided or faulty myths that have been beaten into our heads, I will be happy to have written it. This will all have been worth it if in some way, after having read it, you feel just a little more empowered, prepared, and secure in your decisions, whether you do as I did or do something entirely different. No matter how you choose to navigate your reproductive life, I hope that what guides you is not a panicked reaction to the circumstance you find yourself in but instead is an eyes-wide-open view of the world that allows you to make informed and proactive decisions about your future.

Now get out there and make a few of those big, bold choices we talked about—choices only you can make. Choices you *get* to make. A big, fabulous future is out there waiting for you, entirely yours to shape.

acknowledgments

This book was truly a team effort, and not an easy one for me. I think everyone close to me could attest to the fact this project did not bring out the best in me. The solitary exercise of writing combined with a high-pressure job left me grumpy, irritable, and often unbearable. There were those who literally helped me birth this thing and I want to thank them first, because without them, I would still be on page 1. Katie Arnold, my lifesaver and amazing writing partner who helped shape and create an actual book after my brain dump was complete. Kathy Huck, my editor who put up with an impatient and exhausted first-time author, guiding me through the process. Paul Maroshegyi, my step-dad who was bored enough in retirement to lend me a hand with the initial research. To all the lovely ladies who bravely shared their stories: Kate, Ana, Heather, Heidi, Lauren, Laura, Alison, Amelia, and Victoria, THANK YOU. Without you, this would have been a dull, one-woman show! Bridget Fleming, who shot me for the cover not once but twice, because I make a terrible model (thank you for your patience!) And, of course, the amazing and compassionate doctors who not only help people become parents, but who took the time out of their very important work to help with this book. Dr. Nicole Noyes, who not only contributed the foreword and reviewed the book, but also thought the book was a great idea back when I still wasn't sure I could eke out more than five pages. And last but not least, Dr. Sarah Druckenmiller, who, despite her eighty-hour work weeks as a new doctor, pored over every page to make sure I wrote the best book possible.

Next, there were the two incredible people who inspired me. Whether they knew it or not, they were the wind beneath my very tired wings. Judith Regan took a chance on a girl with a blog, and because I'm in awe of her, I didn't want to let her down. She is the fiercest woman I've ever known and I want to be just like her if I ever grow up! Ernest Lupinacci, aka, my silly Ernielucinni Alfredo with a side of sauce, there are no words. His insane and unfounded belief in me has not only propelled this book to completion, but has made me a better person. THANK YOU.

And of course, there are my friends and family who believed in me and encouraged me even when I was a raging lunatic. First, I have to thank Kate again, because without her, I would never have even considered freezing my eggs. Then there are my brothers who are my rocks, each in their own ways: Chris and Csaba, thank you for being the best brothers anyone could ask for. My sister-in-law Hanna, my cousins and their spouses, Ana, Alex, Endre, Duncan and Brenner, for always asking how things were going. Stella and Matt, two of my biggest cheerleaders. Natasha, who was so supportive from the very beginning and whose lovely dad gave me great advice. Sue, for lending her expertise and guidance. And all of my amazing friends and colleagues at Droga5, especially Jeff, who had to put up with conference calls about eggs and Birth Control 2.0 and me shouting about how HARD IT ALL WAS; Colm, who always had an opinion and was truly interested in the progress I was making; and Duncan, who believes I have another book in me and will be ditching my career in advertising, and who helped me write at least a million iterations of what is now the title of this book. I could go on and on because I have the good fortune of good friends and good family who supported not just my crazy journey with fertility but also the writing of this book. THANK YOU!